First print February 1993

10 9 8 7 6 5 4 3 2 1

Manufactured in the United States of America

Library of Congress Catalog Card Number 92-75757

Where Beauty Touches Me / by Pamela Ferrell of Cornrows & Co.
Includes bibliographical references.
ISBN 0939183-01-3

Cover Photos: Andre Richardson Photography, Washington, D.C.
(202) 529-8682

Cornrows & Co. Publications
5401 14th Street N.W.
Washington, D.C. 20011

Where Beauty Touches Me

Pamela Ferrell
Edited by Carmen Lattimore

Cornrows & Co○ Publication
Washington, D.C. 1993

Dedicated to my beautiful spring girls Amber, Aja, Ebony, Jeanine and Mashon. My gift to you, so that your beauty experience will be culturally stimulating.

Acknowledgments

This book is an expression of my many thanks to the beautiful women in my life who have inspired me to put pen to paper to share their beauty secrets and our discoveries along the way.

Most importantly I thank God for blessing me with good health, a clear mind, and the insight to learn from the many trying and testing experiences of being a beauty renegade. I have learned that the more I share, the more I gain, which has prepared me to complete this beauty book.

Juan Laster, thanks for your sense of humor and laughter. I am indebted to you for running the business as I needed to escape the daily operations. You enabled me the time to finish this book.

I doubt I could have survived my daily struggle with my new Mac computer had it not been for Andre Richardson's guidance and instruction. I will be forever grateful to you for your patience and support when I called you at all hours of the night and day with seemingly endless questions on how to operate my DTP.

Uncle Steve, thank you for driving me to and from Blounts Creek, N.C., so that I could gather words of wisdom from 105 year old Mrs. Belzora Moore.

Mrs. Belzora Moore, Cheryl, Mike, Aunt Patience, Kevin Tripp and family, thank you for the southern hospitality and last minute arrangements to make my visit to Blounts Creek possible. It is evident that our African tradition of hospitality remains in the South. God Bless you all.

With love and respect to my husband, Taalib-Din, I am endeared to you for your relentless support and encouragement in the efforts to make the science of hair braiding a reality in America. You have stood front line with me in the battles and supported me most during my sleepless nights while working on the book.

A very special thanks to my mother and father for always making me feel beautiful... for making my childhood hair care experience a positive one. Never once did you speak negatively about my African characteristics. Your love has shaped me so that I can share this with many women in my life today.

Pamela Ferrell

Foreword

Where Beauty Touches Me is an affirmation, a positive response to any African-American woman whose deep-rooted feelings about her physical features suggest psychological defeat -- the woman who has been conditioned to think that her hair, her countenance, which does not adhere to the Eurocentric ideal, is consequently untouched by beauty and less desirable.

This is a comprehensive guidebook for the whole family, embracing ancient and contemporary African-influenced coiffure and beautification. **Author Pamela Ferrell** begins by taking the reader on a fanciful journey in the voice of a hypocryphal woman who embodies the African beauty aesthetic from the dawn of time to the present. The sojourn begins in East Africa's "Garden of Eden," the earliest known site of original humankind. It continues through time to the earliest documented evidence of ancient Egyptian braided hair styles and beautifying techniques, onward through the lives of the great historical personages and unnamed beauties. These traditional and historical bench marks serve to illustrate the pride with which the African woman has always accepted her inherent features and pursued the enhancement of her appearance.

When the African woman was first captured and transported to America, she began to encounter the Eurocentric beauty standards which still maintain a stronghold today, nearly five hundred years later. A person with a light complexion, blue eyes, keen features, and blonde, straight hair was deemed "good looking" while one with dark skin, full lips, a broad nose, and naturally kinky hair was considered "ugly." **Ms. Ferrell** outlines the accompanying historical suppression of African beauty standards through "corrective cosmetology." She addresses the shocking dangers of chemical straighteners to the body as well as her efforts to champion the natural (chemical-free) beauty aesthetic, met with vehement antagonism by the cosmetology status quo, whose livelihood of straightening kinky hair has yielded a multi-million dollar industry.

The subject of beauty is approached holistically in this book. Demonstrating a profound understanding of the underlying source of beauty, the author acknowledges that physical and spiritual health, together with self-knowledge, are key elements to the superb condition of the hair and scalp. Proper diet, exercise, reduced stress, and a favorable self-concept are inextricably bound to personal appearance. **Ms. Ferrell**, whose goal it is "to improve the mental image inside [her] client's head as well as her outer image which the world sees," seeks to engender a higher level of consciousness toward the beauty potential of her clients and you, the reader.

This book, however, is much more than a philosophical treatise or a Black history lesson. *Where Beauty Touches Me* displays an extensive collection of photographs depicting the range of styles available to the woman who cultivates her hair naturally. Personalized hair and scalp care recommendations are accompanied by recipes for natural hair products you can mix, easily and inexpensively, at home. Those without ready access to a natural stylist should look for the chapters with step-by-step instructions on how to give yourself simply beautiful natural hair styles at home. There are "how-to" instructions on high fashioned braid styles, the care of locks, and varieties of hair extension styles. From washing baby's hair to massaging your man's crowning glory, this book has something for everyone.

Jacquelin Celeste Peters

Jacquelin Celeste Peters *was curator of the critically acclaimed "Music's of Struggle" program at the 1990 Smithsonian Festival of American Folklife. She coordinated the folk festival component of the 1992 National Black Arts Festival. Currently she directs educational programs at the DuSable Museum in Chicago. She authored "Affirming an Ancient Aesthetic," published in the December 1990 edition of* The World & I.

Preface

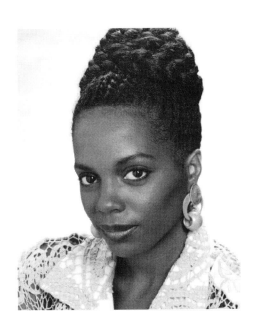

When I lost my job in 1978 for wearing my hair braided, little did I know that my simple attempt to make sure this would never happen to any other woman, would develop a much needed natural hair care industry. The reason for writing this book is to fill the information void for women who choose to wear their hair natural or braided.

My husband and I have diligently worked to bring national attention and change to dress codes that discriminate against African inspired hair styles. We were successful in lobbying the District of Columbia to amended an outdated (1938) cosmetology regulation to include specialty license for the science of hair braiding. The vehement opposition we experienced during our 10 year battle with government bureaucracy was the driving force to make sure this change happened in my lifetime.

Today, major hotels, airlines, corporations, police departments, and the U.S. Army have, as a result, changed their policies. In addition, African-Americans now can create business and educational institutions that promote our culture and the African aestethic.

These small but important changes will make it comfortable for black women to wear their hair in styles that are culturally beautiful and healthy for the hair.

My victory is not having to receive daily phone calls from women nationwide who are fearful of losing their jobs because of their African inspired hair style. The phone calls today are questions concerning the healthy way to care for our hair. I have compiled the numerous questions over the years and tried to answer as many as possible in this beauty book. I hope all women will find something inside that is helpful to their health and beauty evolution.

Pamela Ferrell

Table of Contents   Page

Ground Zero.....

*for me is the Ethiopian soil of the Garden of Eden.
It is dust-colored Eve. And Zipporah crossing the Red Sea. It is Bathsheba conquering the king that slew 10,000. It is Pharoah's daughter and Queen Makeda of Sheba telling the half that's never been told.*

If you had known me then, I was lastingly lovely. The Saharan cornrows designed for me five thousand years ago still grace my head today. In Ancient Africa my braids were symbolic of cultural and social status. You would have known my clan or the Gods I worshiped by the pattern of my braids. Back then, the hairs of my head were numbered. You could count my braids and tell whether I was a princess, queen, or bride. Whatever the sum, you knew I was beautiful.

Sometimes my beauty was accidental. Like the time medicine men applied salves to my eye lids, lashes , and brows; dusting them with powdered lead, copper, or anything else to protect and sooth me from the Egyptian sun. My colored eyes were so alluring to the men that this began a cosmetics industry.

Other times I was incidentally lovely with pellets of sweet spices, honey, and anti-gum freshening my breath. And henna juice stain-ing my fingernails and toenails. Elaborate wigs of natural hair, sheep's wool, and plant fibers were fashioned to protect me from the sun. Back then I admired myself, my earrings and strings of precious beads in polished copper mirrors specially crafted to reflect my beauty.

I was naturally beautiful. So much that it caused me much pain. My body was carved with crystal splinters to appease the Gods. Rites of passage were etched into my skin in designs of raised ridges and dots. I was a living language written in beauty. Back then I was adorned in truth. You could read my markings and know the strength of my character. You could trace my history on the contours of my cheeks. If you had known me back then, I could have let you feel each evolution as you touched the place where beau-ty touches me.

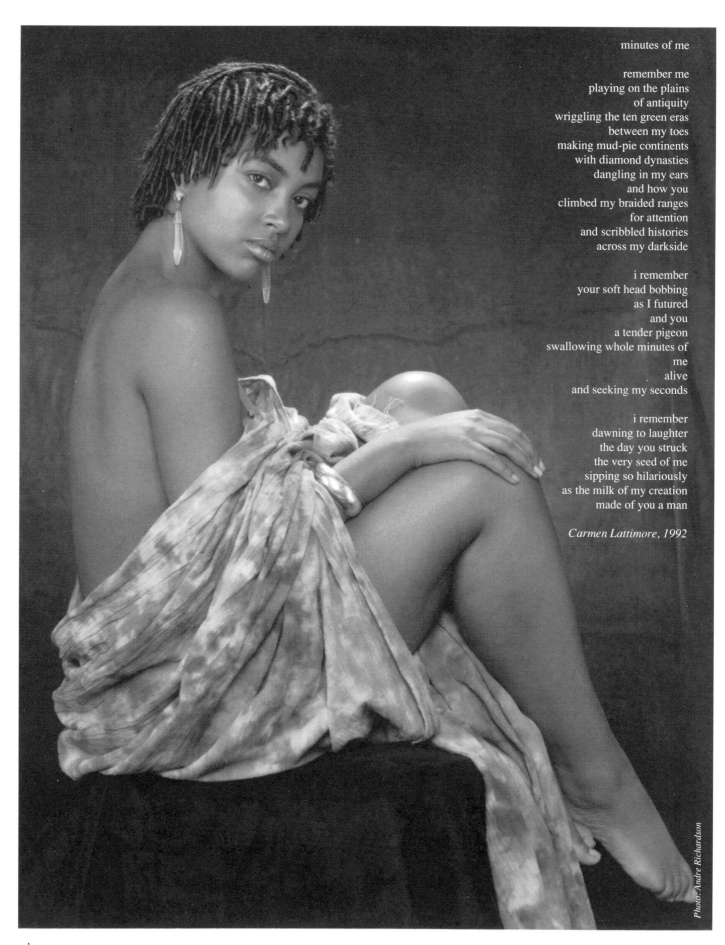

minutes of me

remember me
playing on the plains
of antiquity
wriggling the ten green eras
between my toes
making mud-pie continents
with diamond dynasties
dangling in my ears
and how you
climbed my braided ranges
for attention
and scribbled histories
across my darkside

i remember
your soft head bobbing
as I futured
and you
a tender pigeon
swallowing whole minutes of
me
alive
and seeking my seconds

i remember
dawning to laughter
the day you struck
the very seed of me
sipping so hilariously
as the milk of my creation
made of you a man

Carmen Lattimore, 1992

xiv

1
History ....From Darkness to Light

From Darkness to Light

Things are different for the American black woman. How she knows herself today is reflected in her understanding of the past. Since the beauty standard here is still European, we must hold onto what we are because we can never be what we are not. Let us observe the history of our female beauty legends for they are the depositors of our beauty ideals. Cultivation of physical beauty has been one of great pain in the African-American experience, however, we must regenerate our true beauty aesthetic.

.

THE COSMETIC CONSPIRACY

Corrective Cosmetology

When Africans arrived to the "New World" America, the beautification and appreciation of their thick, natural hair ended. Africans, who were used to skillfully crafted combs made of fine woods and ivory, were subjected to slave living conditions which lacked even the barest grooming utensils and cosmetics for black hair and skin. And, in addition to the hostile physical environment, a psychologically defeating ideal of beauty was forced upon the Africans in America. For the first time black people were made to feel ugly and inferior as they were compared with the physiognomy of the Europeans, who dominated the "New World." Just as black skin was considered on the negative side opposite white beauty, wooly, curly hair was the least desirable as it was compared to straight blond hair. Consequently, black people learned to hate their complexion and the texture of their natural hair.

The Battle of the Naps

All beauty regiments for black hair were designed with the original intent of hiding or "correcting" its nappy condition. Thus, pomades and the straightening comb became a dynamic duo in the hands of a beautician whose job was to eliminate the natural nap of the black woman's hair at any cost. She waged valiant warfare against her arch enemies; water and perspiration, which invariably caused her straightened hair to revert back to its natural, nappy state. For this reason, many black women disdained athletics (especially swimming) lest they "sweat" their straightened hair out. And, needless to say, this endless and futile war with nature fattened the pockets of the black beautician.

Black women were in search of a permanent solution to this problem, and it was finally offered to them in the 1940s in the form of lye-based chemical processors. And once again the cosmetics industry profited richly.

In the 1960s, it took an act of Congress and a militant black power movement to cause black women to try a "fad" hair style called the Afro. For the first time, many black women learned to enjoy the splendid luxury of their natural hair. In fact, even white women began to address their beautcian for a permanent that would add nap and kink to their hair. Pride in the black heritage began to overturn centuries of shame and fear of our black identity. Unfortunately, however, many black cosmetologist suffered financial losses because the Afro hair style required little or no professional maintenance. And for the first time black people were able to pocket the money that had been financing the "corrective" beauty culture.

Preventive Cosmetology

In the United States the "fads" of natural hair and braided styles have been violently opposed by an economy which has made millions of dollars promoting a mentality among black people that their natural hair is wrong or ugly. The products and processes of the American cosmetology industry imply that somehow God made a mistake, and black people were born with bad hair. Therefore, they need to buy something or pay somebody to help them achieve a good hair texture.

With all of the gels, glues, relaxers, and spritzers on the American shelves ready to enforce every chemically straightened strand of hair, a natural hair stylist like myself is almost an affront to this industrial conspiracy to prevent the Afro or anything close to it from raising its "ugly" head in America again. Whether this preventive cosmetology is racially or greed motivated is not the issue. My deepest concern is for the damage this hype and frenzy over straight hair has done to the black female's hair follicle.

I believe that the false accusation by the cosmetology industry that black hair does not grow long is a direct result of the irresponsible destruction of our natural hair by heat and chemical warfare.

BEAUTY IS GROWING

I do not agree with the saying that "beauty is skin deep." I believe that beauty begins within-- in the mind, spirit and heart of a woman. How she feels about herself from the inside radiates on the outside of her countenance. Therefore, it is always my goal as a cosmetologist to improve the mental image inside my client's head as well as her outer image which the world sees. I heartily agree that "beauty is in the eye of the beholder," but it must be the woman herself who first beholds herself as beautiful.

The Mende women of Africa see beauty simply as something growing. Growth is the focus of this book, not only the healthy growth of natural hair, but the evolution of girl to woman. From ignorance to full knowledge of self as beautiful. Growing as a beautician has meant learning my clientele, understanding the outer-pressures of their society and the inner-pressures of fear and insecurity. It has meant expanding their horizons to understand that the world did not originate in Europe, and that original beauty was not blonde but was, in fact, women of color.

THERAPEUTIC COSMETOLOGY

Women usually come to my salon with a problem. Their hair has been damaged by abusive heat and chemical treatments, or they desire a style which cannot be achieved with their natural hair. They have either suffered some degree of hair loss and want to cover up the problem with hair extensions, or they desire a weave of long hair to lengthen their own shorter hair. Many times their problem is deeper than a band-aid can hide. Because they have never gotten to know themselves as beautiful, and they had no respect for their natural hair, they consequently permitted the beautician to sacrifice their hair growth and good health for the sake of social acceptability and style.

It is always my objective to help my clients understand the beauty that is inherently their own-- the same black beauty which has no rival in history except in this country. I try to help my clients know the roots of their own beautiful hair.

Experiencing her natural beauty can be an ecstatic thing for a woman. It is exciting for me to witness the evolution of an insecure, damaged woman into a natural beauty. Something marvelous occurs when she realizes that she was born beautiful and that her natural hair is soft, manageable, and alluring. Beauty happens on the inside of this woman. She radiates a peaceful confidence that she didn't have before. Everybody loves a beautiful thing, and these women begin to love themselves in a way that they never had before.

Because I always have this goal at heart, my responses to my clients may differ from other hair stylists. I want to know up front what they want from me because they may want something that I can't give them. They may want me to lie to them and tell them that they'd look lovely with hip length blond hair, when I know they would not. It is not my intention to just sit something on top of a client's head for a price. If I know that her request or expectations are absurd, impractical, or detrimental, I will try to raise her level of consciousness about her potential as a beautiful black woman. I will show her alternate hair styles, and diagnose her beauty attributes beginning with her age, facial features, and career status. I will try to understand both her internal and external pressures. Together we will create a look for her that will make her feel good about herself first and appeal to her society second. It is my desire to strengthen her self-esteem as well as her hair texture.

If I were to generalize, there are six types of women who come into my salon today: *Natural Beauty, Ms. Thang, Misfitted, Un-Made, Self-Hater and Tom-Boy.* Even though women are very different in their profiles, each type can be described as best or worst.

The Natural Beauty

Most women have the potential to be a natural beauty. This woman radiates calmness and serenity. She is motherly without being matronly. She is admired for both her physical beauty and her inner spirit. This woman gets more beautiful with time.

She was usually nurtured in a loving environment of supportive men and women who assured her early in life of the value of beauty. She understands that her beauty is not to be compared to others, but simply shared with all. She is hygienically clean. She has clear skin and appropriate make-up. Her features are proportional. Her eyes are bright and sparkle with vitality. Her hair is clean, full-bodied, and growing; her hair style simple. She is never overdone.

The natural beauty understands beauty. She exercises, eats well, and guards her spiritual well-being. Although natural beauties have a definite sense of style, some may not be fully evolved in realizing their full potential. I can be most creative with this easy client because she is secure, open to ideas, and needs little or no major changes in appearance.

Best: The key word is "simplicity." She is simply beautiful, and she already understands it.

Worst: She is too plain and needs a touch of stylized direction to reach her peak potential.

Ms. Thang

This woman is trying to bloom. She strives to keep up with the ever changing trends while having no definite style of her own. If it looks good on the model in the magazine and she likes it, she wants it (even if it will look terrible on her).

Someone has told this woman that she is beautiful, and she has blindly accepted it as fact. Such a presumption makes her over-confident, bordering on arrogant. Her skin reflects her cavalier attitude. Her hair condition betrays the fact that she has spent more time and money on style than care. She has colored her hair one week, permed it the next, and wants extensions and re-color today. If the price tag were the only obstacle, Ms. Thang would find a way to pay for the style of her choice. One client said to me, "I'd pay $100,000 to get rid of my nappy hair." Probably in her lifetime this Ms. Thang will spend more than that, all in trying to become something she is not.

Marjorie is a Ms. Thang. She is a "wanna bee" model with an extensive personal wardrobe. Because she feels she is always in the public eye, her make-up and fashions are often avant-garde and exaggerated. For instance, during the winter Marjorie will actually dye her hair to match her fur coat. And her eyelashes are as long as her designer fingernails. I once gave her hip length braids that took twenty hours to complete. Even though she may look extreme she will not abuse her good looks. She tries to eat well and gets plenty of exercise. Marjorie is beautiful to behold, but she is definitely not a natural beauty.

I try to meet Ms. Thang half way by encouraging her to focus on enhancing her own good features without trying to look like another woman. I suggest a "healthy" high fashion style that will allow her hair to rest. For example, if her hair is damaged, thin, and not full enough to create one of her wish-styles, I use an enhancer like hair extensions to give her the style while protecting her natural hair.

Ms. Thang is usually open to change if she likes and trusts her beauty consultant, and she will attempt to be naturally attractive if it is fashionably correct.

Best: Fashionably chic, but a little too overdone. Accessories may be bordering on gaudiness, and her hair style is usually garish.

Worst: Excessive make-up, frills, and hair style cause her to look vulgar and cheap -- almost like a harlot.

The Misfitted

This woman has no place to be herself. For economic and/or social purpose she has been forced to fit into roles, styles, and an environment not necessarily of her choosing. She may feel constricted and repressed without even knowing it. She appears stiff and uncomfortable in her tailored suit or high heeled shoes. Everything about her looks too large, too small, or out dated because she has cultivated her self-image from a magazine or shopper's catalog. Her style is controlled by her society, whether it be her parents, spouse, career, or religion.

The salon is almost like a psychiatrist's office for the misfitted client. She must be handled with kid gloves because she is so adamant in her opinions. Somewhere in her past conditioning, she was made to believe that she was not acceptable unless she dressed a certain way or had a certain kind of hair. Often the misfitted woman will not waver on that un-natural image of herself.

With this client only gradual progress is possible because I must first gain enough trust to attempt even minor changes in her mental attitude and style. She is the beauticians biggest challenge. In fact, you cannot call yourself an "expert" in the field until you have successfully assisted one of these clients to better understand who they are when they look in the mirror. The misfitted woman has taught me patience and has helped me evolve as a hair care professional.

She is usually meek but has a heart of gold. When she comes to our salon she is extremely inquisitive about our techniques and products, but she invariably selects a style that would be unflattering. She pretends that she wants to change her image but will confusingly refuse to do so. She will show me a photo or a wig of the style she wants and expects that I duplicate it strand for strand on her head. What is worse, sometimes she expects the style to stay perfectly in place until her next appointment at the salon. Janece was like that. When she came in for a hair weave, she was wearing an enormous wig that reminded me of Marie Antoinette in the 18th century . Her bangs were so long and heavy that I could barely see her nose.

No matter how long this woman comes to me (one or ten years) she will not change her style. She is constantly struggling for perfection. This woman is usually intimidated by her own hair and does not know how to style it herself.

Despite her shortcomings, she is a loyal client, even though she often appears to be unhappy. Her beautician is just like her hair style -- permanent and there for life. She will usually not follow her beautician's advice and often has to admit her mistakes later. And interestingly so, this woman will not abuse her natural hair.

She just requires time, patience and constant assurance. She is a bruised rose who never had the chance to evolve into a natural beauty. I can only continue to nurture this flower with great gratitude, and though her petals will never change, they will also never wither.

Best: She is satisfied that she has achieved the image she desires. She

3

will maintain her style even if it is not the most flattering for her.

Worst: Incapable of fitting her self-image, she looks unmanageable, outdated, and grotesque. She is often emotionally unhappy with herself.

The Un-Made Woman

This woman does not pay attention to the detail of her beauty. She is tiredly plain, almost as if she is incomplete. She seems to be more comfortable than the misfitted because she does not feel the need or pressure to please anyone with her beauty. She lacks the artistic eye to create a pleasant image of herself and the motivation to try. The un-made woman is inclined to "let herself go" at times. She does not have a beauty glow and she has low self-esteem. There is a dullness in her personality, complexion, and her appearance. Often this woman has poor health and lacks the energy to care for herself. It is common to see the un-made woman with a drug addiction or alcohol dependency problem.

Best: She is very plain, neat, clean, and could go un-noticed. There is nothing interesting about her appearance.

Worst: She is a slovenly woman. She is a mess, an eye sore to look at. Trifling, lazy, and unclean. Her make-up is rushed; her hair soiled and uncombed, her nails are dirty, and polish is chipped; and her teeth may be rotten. This woman does not take any time to care for herself.

The Self-Hater

This woman is often the true bi-product of the negativity of American racism within the black community. She is usually a very attractive woman who has been taught to dislike some or all aspects of her beauty. During her childhood, people may have made unkind remarks about her physical features, or she may have been emotionally abused. Whatever the cause, the result is a woman who feels totally unpretty. She uses skin lightener or darkener. She changes the color of her eyes (blue or green) and hair (blonde) to the extreme. She is constantly removing or adding some adornment to her body, even though doing so may be harmful to her health.

In this phase there are white women who desire all the attributes of African women: tan skin, plump lips, round buttocks, thick curly hair. And there are black women who strive to look European: straight hair, keen nose, no hips, and light skin. All races have self-haters.

The philosophy of the self-hater is, "Why live through life not liking the woman in the mirror? I'd rather be beautiful by any way possible." Her life evolves around creating herself opposite to what she is naturally. She is therefore cursed with striving to meet certain beauty standards that are not her own. This makes her insecure and unstable in her beauty decisions.

Mirian was a self-hater when I first met her. When she came to the salon her brittle blond hair was pulled back in a rubber band. She had dark eyebrows drawn above her blue eye shadow. She wore black pencil liner around her lips attempting to make them look smaller. Many of her bright fingernail tips were broken off, and her white blouse was stretched so tight around her breasts that her black bra peeped through the buttonholes. Such a woman needs positive assurance that she is beautiful without all the fuss. She must be re-conditioned to believe that her natural beauty is okay and sufficient. Her beauty salon experience should be a relaxing one where she can shed some of her negative baggage.

Best: She only verbalizes her dislike of her self-image. She feels she can not do better so she negates her African beauty as well as the beauty of others in that image.

Worst: She is self mutilating. She will do things that are harmful to her health for the sake of re-creating her beauty... unnecessary plastic surgery, skin bleaching, chemically over processing the hair, unhealthy diet, and destructive life style.

The Tom-Boy

This woman would be closer to the natural beauty if only she cared enough about her femininity. She spends minimal time primping and grooming herself. Her mannerisms are hard and masculine. Her attitude is that if the shower does not take care of it, nothing will. She usually wears hats or scarves in order to do little or nothing to her hair. To look at her she appears lazy, but that is not the case. She simply prefers not to invest much in something that could bring her more attention than she would like to have. She is not comfortable with frills, lace, or bows. This female may have been of the other gender in her past life. Comfort is the most important thing for this woman. I would suggest to the Tom-Boy female, the fashion of tailored wear with a feminine touch in the style design and colors. Her hair style should be soft and flowing with a neat shape and low maintenance for her easy, low-key style.

Best: She is attractive and athletically inclined. She is fresh looking, exercises, and eats well.

Worst: Her style emulates a man. Her behavior and appearance are stiff and macho. She is a sloppy dresser and gives little attention to her overall feminine appearance.

2

The Garden of Beauty Evolution

BEAUTY EVOLUTION

From birth her body is expected to grow because growth depicts life. If a woman learns to value her hair and body she can minimize many of her beauty ills. She will take special care not to deprive her body of nutrition and its life giving elements. As a reward, she should expect strong, growing, beautiful hair.

In Western Africa, "big hair," "much hair" is considered a distinctly feminine trait. In the Mende nation,

such hair is praised as " kpotongo," meaning "it is much, abundant, plentiful." The root word, "kpoto," is often used to describe fruits on a tree, rice, and other growing things. "Kpoto," meaning long and thick, denotes hair that grows like a farm or forest. These ideas about hair reinforce the Mende identification of women with the Great Mother Earth, the female principle of God Almighty. Trees, plants, shrubs, vines, bushes, flowers, herbs-- verdure is "hair" on the head of Earth Mother, just as the hair on the head of a woman is like her flora, her special environment, for foliage.

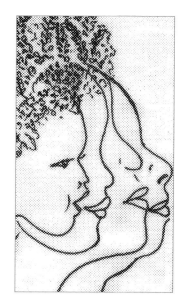

Plants and human hair have the same capacity of growth and increase. A woman with long, thick hair demonstrates the life-force, the multiplying power of profusion, prosperity, a "green thumb" for raising bountiful farms and many healthy children. [1]

To me a woman's hair is like a garden of flowers which comes in all varieties of colors and shapes. The hair shaft which is above the scalp can be compared to leaves and petals. The hair below the scalp would be the roots, the foundation of the garden. The hair root is embedded in a pocket-like hole called the follicle. At the end of a follicle is a bulb that is connected to the blood vessels.

The blood stream carries nutrients directly to the hair root.

Therefore, any adversities in the blood have a like effect on the hair growth and its condition. For this reason, traces of all chemicals, medications, and drugs administered to a person can be found in the hair.

Just as poisonous chemicals adversely affect the natural soil, heavy petroleum, greases, and synthetic oils placed on the scalp can clog the pores and follicles and thereby suffocate the roots of the hair. Also harsh chemicals, such as lye-based relaxer and curly perms, can burn the scalp, and the resultant scar tissue will prevent hair growth.

In the same way that the climate affects the growth of plants, a woman's circumstances and emotional environment can affect her diet and thus her hair. Stress, hormonal conditions, an ailing nervous system, and "the change of life" can all cause hair thinning and baldness.

GROWING SEASONS

Like gardens, hair grows in seasons. As a female matures from infancy to adulthood, the climate of her lifestyle and temperament can be contrasted with the growing seasons of a garden. Just as flowers grow during certain months in the spring and summer, so does a female's evolution.

_____ _1_
Radiance from the Waters, Sylvia Ardyn Boone, Yale Publications.

Spring

From birth to age 24, a woman is in the spring of her life. She is born ready to be molded. Her beauty ideals are formed largely by her sensual experiences. What she sees, feels, and hears. A mother's touch should be kind and gentle during this season. A mother must teach the early spring female to nurture and cherish her health and beauty. Hair is usually virgin and fragile during this time of evolution. It should not be pulled in too tight braids, rubber bands, or barretts which can cause traction Alopecia (premature hair loss around the hairline). The spring female will begin to develop confidence and self-esteem. Through learning to love herself, she will learn to appreciate the beauty of others without making negative comparisons.

All too soon, the protective and strengthening beauty regiments of childhood give way to the experimentation and flamboyance of the adolescent and teen years. The female becomes very conscious of her appearance during this season, as she attempts to beautify and adorn herself. By then the wise spring female's hair is healthy and sturdy, and good grooming and hygiene habits have been formed. During mid-to-late spring, hair becomes a full-bloom cascade. And of course, the bees (boys) begin to buzz around her during this season!

Length, vitality and strength of strand are important during the high school and college years. Because the body and hair are in their most rapid growing stage during this season, the spring diet should be simple and purely natural. But all too often a large part of the high school and college student's diet consists of processed fast foods, junk snacks, and carbonated beverages.

The special problems of this season are complicated by parents who teach one thing and do another. A young lady who is compelled to "bathe and eat right" by a mother who is unkempt and overweight herself or who suggests that her daughter's African features need to be "fixed" will suffer from insecurity and confusion during this season. Many young women are mentally and emotionally scarred during their teens by parents who do not understand this developmental stage. This is the time for the female to bud and unfold, not to be bruised before she reaches the full bloom of summer.

Summer

From ages 25 to 49 a woman's beauty yields gracefully to the demands of increasing dimension. This is the season of display and mating. She will be noticed for her evolution into a whole woman. However, if the spring was not fertile, the summer woman will be a late-bloomer, as she tries to play catch-up during her twenties. The foliage of summer hair should be rich and luxurious. Styles should be easy to manage and cost efficient for mothers with small children, chic and crisp for the working and professional woman. Unfortunately, early summer hair styles may reflect an attempt to make this beauty look older than she is. Continuing in this vain will cause the fickle summer woman to try too much too soon as she creates and recreates her sensual, career and self-image. Her quest to be a "perfect 10" can be extremely devastating for her hair as she perms, curls, colors, cuts, and otherwise over-processes her hair.

Emotional disorders or "bad nerves" from job, marriage, and parenting pressures often complicate this season's growth by causing personal beauty care neglect. A negative self-perspective resulting from loss of mate or job or being told she's too young or too old to attain her goals adversely affects her self-esteem. The summer woman's diet, hormones, and , medications during pregnancy and childbearing also have a profound impact on hair growth and health.

It is important that she enter the intensity of summer season totally secure and realistically expectant of more responsibility, discipline, and care. Such a woman will prosper into full growth during this most productive season. She will rise to master the consuming demands of the career mother. By applying a beauty regiment to enhance and protect the natural beauty of her hair, she will survive the locusts and cankers of environmental frustration which are the greatest culprits to her growth. Her beauty will ripen into whole and abundant fruit for the coming harvest.

Autumn

The reaping years from age 50-75, this truly beautiful woman is gathering her accomplishments and glorying in her gains. She is preparing for a full harvest in every aspect of her life. But she has changed from the diligent, busy caterpillar of summer into a wonderful butterfly ready for new horizons. Her hair styles reflect her new confidence. They are colorful, light and comfortable. Free now from the cares of summer, she is expensive and indulgent in her beauty regiment. She has learned her body. Her diet is natural and full of nutrients and fiber. She alternates relaxation with long walks in the fresh air and pleasurable exercise. She is prepared for the onset of "the change of life." She is promoted to mother of the bride and grandmother in the relationships. In her career, she has risen to the level of experienced authority. She is now the confident assessor and not the assessed.

But, if the fall woman has suffered a hard, barren summer, she may enter the season in poor emotional and physical health. Instead of the harvest, she may be mourning an unmanageable, overgrown, or failed crop. Having neglected her health and beauty for the rigors of an unsuccessful life plan, she may feel discouraged. She feels she is too old to be beautiful, and it is too late to try again. Her hair may be brittle, broken, and balding. She may have a chronic physical ailments like high blood pressure or arthritis.

In this case, autumn is her season to take emergency action to salvage and preserve her beauty assets. Such a woman needs a new attitude. She must practice drastic "me first" measures where her physical and mental well-being are concerned. A good doctor and expert hair care stylist can help her correct some things, but she must also have positive emotional and spiritual support. As her physical body prepares for the quiet storm of winter, her inner woman must be strengthened to sustain a peaceful, self-appreciating countenance.

Autumn is simply the spring of winter. This woman deserves to look and feel good. She does not slow down, she sets her cruise-control.

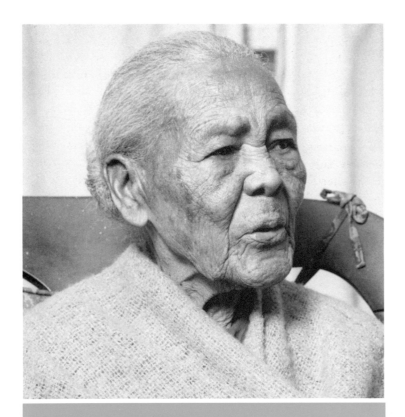

Mrs. Belzora Moore of Blounts Creek, N.C., is a true winter woman, age 105. Born August 21, 1887--- she is still enjoying her final season.

Winter

During the cultivated, restful period from year 76 on, a woman comes of age. These are her smiling years. Her laugh lines are well travelled. Her beauty has been bundled, ribboned, and brought indoors for company. She is like silk flowers and potpourri. Her sterling silver hair is an expensive centerpiece. Her presence is an emblem of honor accentuating every environment. Now she influences and changes others more than she is changed herself.

Both her body and her hair have changed. They are fine and fragile like china. This is her time for balance, peace, and a controlled, harmonious environment. Her beauty styles are gentle and low-impact. Her hair should be allowed to grow undisturbed and as well as it pleases. Free temples and neat chignons are this woman. Her diet should be light and easy to digest, incorporating plenty of herbs and fresh fruits and vegetables.

She is a gift woman, full of surprises and delights for the young. Winter is her season as she celebrates wrapped victories with the coming and going younger women. She has much wisdom to share. Just as the snow covers and protects the ground for the next spring, her life stories prepare and protect all who come for her blessings.

It is always sad for me to see worn and weathered winter women. During this time women should not be worried about balding. They should not feel neglected. In their youth these women were nurtured by a generation of caring beauticians who were often trusted friends. So many winter women feel betrayed by the impersonal chemical cosmetology of today. Their fine, thinning hair should not be sacrificed for the sake of beauty. Mama Nelson initially came to my salon to buy very expensive extensions to match her silver-white hair. She returned two days later in tears because her braided hair style

7

was very unattractive, and she had a church program to attend. She had been left emotionally distraught by an insensitive, inexperienced hair braider. Because they are accustomed to beauticians that befriend and grow with them, they often fall prey to the mercenary practitioner. Mama Nelson was so hurt by this experience that I had to work harder to restore her broken spirit than I did on her new hair style. We got her off to her church program with a smile, but this experience left a lasting impression on me.

Daughters, be cautious about recommending younger beauticians or inexperienced hair braiders to your mother and grandmothers. Cosmetology is generally a young woman's business, and we cannot afford to overlook the needs of women who are in their winter season for the sake of convenience and expense. For the senior women in our lives, a hair care professional should be the equivalent of an expert gift wrapper. Her main objective should be to package this exquisite present for grateful and awaiting recipients -- women in the early seasons.

In the haste of the younger season's busy lifestyle, she must take time to sit down and communicate with elder women, not only is this a moment to receive valuable information, but it is the perfect stress relief in this time of rush.

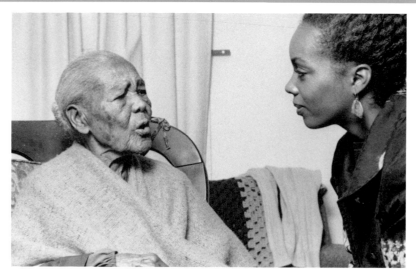

I was blessed to have the company of several winter women who shared their life secrets with me. Ninty-eight year old grandma Stewart (Mrs. Edith Stewart of Marvel, Arkansas Feb. 26, 1894 - Oct. 30, 1992), whom I have known for seven years, passed one month after our woman-to-woman beauty chat. Her words of wisdom to me were : *Think pleasant thoughts, surround yourself with good people; eat fresh fruits and vegetables for good health , and eat a handful of raw sunflower seeds a day for good eyesight. To her, beauty is within a person; intelligence is beautiful. To live a long, healthy life keep your mind active and occupied.*

Mrs. Belzora (above), 105 years old, says she worked from age nine to age seventy and she believes a little hard work will not hurt a woman. She remembers, as a child, her mother wrapping her hair with black thread to keep it healthy and soft. On special outings her mother would loosen the wrapped hair and put a bow on it. She has never used chemicals in her hair, and she never pressed her children's hair (four girls). For diet she tells younger women to pay attention to their systems. If what you eat does not feel good to your system (body), do not eat it. Her diet consists of fresh fruits , vegetables, and no red meat. She recommends to younger woman to preserve your health and beauty *"Listen to good people, go to church , and follow the good book."*

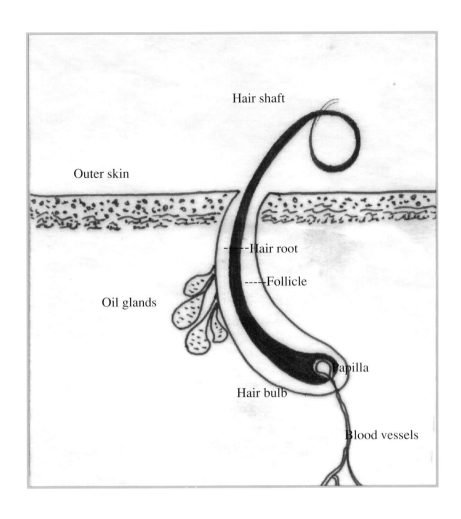

Hair shaft

Outer skin

Hair root

Follicle

Oil glands

Papilla

Hair bulb

Blood vessels

THE HAIR......

The composition of hair varies based on the hair type, one's age, sex, origin, and hair color. Hair is composed of oxygen, hydrogen, carbon, nitrogen, sulfur, and phosphorus. It is a hard fiber protein known as keratin. The average person's hair grows 1/2" per month and is 4-5% sulfur. Sulfur is an element of protein. The formation of hair begins with the digestion of high quality proteins in the diet.

**Good hair** is growing hair that has good elasticity, porosity, and texture.

**Bad hair** is no hair! or hair that is damaged, dry , and slow growing.

Hair shaft-- the part of hair that extends above the skin.

Hair root-- the part of hair that is below the scalp.

Follicle-- A hole that holds the hair root.

Oil Glands-- Sacs that produce sebum, which keeps the hair naturally lubricated and supple.

Papilla-- receives the rich blood and nerve supply which contribute to its growth.

Bulb--the lower part of the hair root which covers the papilla.

Blood vessels-- transport the nutrients to the hair papilla.

LACK OF KNOWLEDGE is the greatest cause of hair problems. Hair in these modern times is worse than in the past because of the availability of products and harmful applications by untrained and unthinking people. Having a good knowledge of your hair and how it relates to the overall health is important.

Your hair on the head serves two purposes: **1.** protection, to shield the head from injury and the external elements **2.** adornment for pleasure. The fundamental reason women beautify their hair is to look and feel good. Unfortunately, women have placed more value on looking good than they have on taking care of their hair and body. How you treat your hair and your body is ultimately reflected by your mental health.

MENTAL HEALTH is a clear, focused, and intelligent mind; a positive perspective about yourself, your culture, and life in general. The mind puts things into action. We are what we think.

Because more and more women have created a superwoman lifestyle, it is common to see women suffering from mental fatigue, low self-esteem, and depression, therefore neglecting their diet and ignoring their beauty needs. A woman's mental attitude affects how she values herself and ultimately how she takes care of herself. As a hair stylist, I see women when they are feeling inadequate, and at a vulnerable point to either neglect their beauty care or abuse themselves in trying to make up for the inadequacy.

I encourage them to develop a positive mental outlook since this is paramount to good health and happiness. The mind becomes a healing agent when women develop the ability to visualize complete health and physical well-being. For example, if you see yourself as being overworked and exhausted, not having the energy to groom yourself, you will continue to live that existence you visualize and apply. A different view naturally creates a different self. It is helpful for women to begin to re-examine their lives and find a discipline such as prayer, self-dialogue, or meditation. These disciplines can enable you to adopt a different mental attitude. Healthy hair and a healthy body are manifestations of good mental health. The mind is what shapes active beauty ideals. For example, if you believe that you are ugly, the negative would be to put that idea into action and use that as a fulfilling goal to tell yourself " I am not worthy of making myself beautiful because I have no control over my looks." The positive mental response would be to say to oneself, "I like the way I look; I am uniquely attractive, and I will do the necessary things to maintain my health and beauty."

A healthy mental outlook is having peace, balance and a sense of control of your life.

Spiritual Health is understanding your purpose in the spirit life; past and present-- who you are, where you come from (your ancestors), and your purpose here in the metaphysical life. Having good spiritual health creates a sense of balance, truth, and faith in yourself and God. Developing a higher spiritual understanding gives you the inner state of clarity, you need to become a more centered person. Meditation and prayer are ways to nurture and extend your spiritual health. Once you are spiritually enriched, you will begin to take control of your mental and physical well-being.

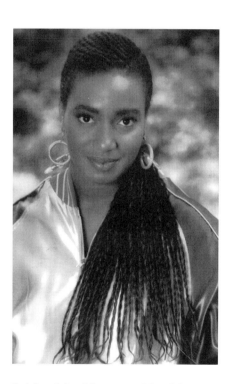

Spiritual health, mental health, good hygiene, exercise, fresh air, sun shine and a nutritious diet are the ingredients for self-preservation

HOW DOES YOUR DIET AFFECT YOUR HAIR GROWTH?

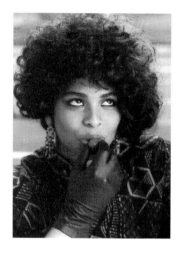

To develop a clear understanding about your healthy hair, its life cycle and what can stimulate its growth, you must fully appreciate the human anatomy--more specifically your body. Hair growth is not independent of your nervous, excretory, lymph, and blood systems. Healthy hair growth relies on internal nourishment received by means of the blood vessels. There has been no medical evidence to suggest that hair can receive its nourishment through "hair foods" pomades, gels, or other hair products.

The hair is nourished by small blood vessels that are attached to the hair bulb at the root of the hair. Quite naturally, in order to assure good quality blood to the hair, you must supply your body with the proper nutrients, vitamins, minerals, proteins, and trace elements that are found in the foods you eat. A healthy diet should consist of 60%

raw fresh fruits and vegetables every day (no canned or frozen).

FRUITS and VEGETABLES

Apples	Asparagus
Apricots	Beans
Avocados	Beets & tops
Bananas	Broccoli
Berries	Cabbage
Cherries	Celery
Carrots	Cauliflower
Currants	Chard
Dates	Chicory
Figs	Chives
Grapes	Collards
Grapefruit	Cucumbers
Lemons, ripe	Dandelion
Kiwi	Dulse
Limes	Eggplant
Mangoes	Garlic
Melons, all	Greens
Nectarines	Kale
Oranges	Legume
Papaya	Lettuce
Peaches	Mushrooms
Pears	Onions
Plums	Okra
Pineapples	Parsley
Pomegranates	Pepper
Prunes	Potatoes
Raisins	Pumpkin
Tangerines	Sprouts
Tomatoes	Squash
	Turnips
	Soybeans
	Spinach
	Watercress
	Water chestnuts

DAILY SERVING FOR A GOOD DIET

* **Two servings of fresh fruit** daily, best eaten at breakfast.

***Six servings of vegetables per day.** (Raw salads include many vegetables) A raw salad with lunch and dinner is a good practice.

* **One serving of a starch** (baked potato, squash, rice, cereal, pasta, grains, peas, bread)

* **One serving of a protein** (fish, beans, cheese, eggs, tofu, seeds, poultry)

* **Up to 7 (8 oz.) glasses of liquid.** (Water, raw juices, soy milks, lemonade, herbal teas) **AVOID COFFEE, SODA, ALCOHOL, CAFFEINE TEAS**

AVOID CONSUMING FATS or HYDROGENATED OILS: Butter, fat meats, lard, margarine, cream, tallow.

For cooking and salad dressings USE COLD PRESSED OILS: Nut oils, olive oil, soy oil, safflower oil, sunflower oil, sesame oil.

AVOID WHITE PROCESSED SUGAR: candy, sugar substitutes, chocolates, pastries.

USE IN MODERATION AS A SWEETENER: Raw honey, maple syrup, molasses, date sugar, raw sugar.

ESSENTIAL ELEMENTS REQUIRED FOR THE NUTRITION OF (WO)MAN

Major Mineral Elements:
Calcium

Iodine

Potassium

Chlorine

Magnesium

Silicon

Fluorine

Manganese

Sodium

Iron

Phosphorus

Sulphur

Air Elements:
Carbon

Oxygen

Hydrogen

Nitrogen

Elements found in Hair:
Carbon

Oxygen

Phosphorus

Hydrogen

Nitrogen

Sulphur

SPECIAL HERBS AND VITAMINS THAT HELP HEALTHY HAIR GROWTH:

Dulse--it can be used to replace salt; high in iodine, minerals, and vitamins needed for hair growth.

Horsetail--- use as a tea or capsule; helps to stop falling hair.

Sage---use as a tea, oil, or rinse for the scalp; an astringent for the scalp, stimulates hair growth.

Rosemary---helpful hair rinse and oil for baldness, strengthens the hair.

Basil oil--helps to loosen hardened sebum on the scalp and in the follicle.

Nettle--use as a hair rinse, antiseptic; helps baldness,and dandruff problems.

Kelp---sea vegetable, rich in iodine, calcium, sulphur, and silicon; promotes overall health of glands, thyroid which stimulates the metabolism for healthy hair growth.

Vitamin C--aids in improving scalp circulation, builds the body immune system which protects against free-radicals, vaginal dryness, and depression.

Vitamin B Complex---B vitamins are important for hair growth.

Vitamin E--- Increases oxygen intake, which improve circulation to the scalp. Increases the production of hormones, relieves hot flashes and dryness in the vagina.

Black cohosh-- contains a natural estrogen (the estrogen levels drop during menopause); helps to control hot flashes.

Licorice root-- contains natural estrogen, increases energy.

Calcium & Magnesium chelate--relieves nervousness and irritability.

Potassium-- helps to control heavy perspiring.

Gota Kola-- relieves hot flashes, vaginal dryness, and depression.

Iodine--a trace mineral which can be found in sea food and sea vegetables. It helps to produce thyroxine for the proper function of the thyroid gland.

Menopause

"The Change of Life"

This is the time in a woman's life when the menstrual period stops. The *change of life* usually happens to the late Summer / early Autumn woman (age 40-50). Although every woman is affected differently, most experience similar symptoms. I find it important for me to talk to the woman that is experiencing this phase of her life because the discomforts she will have affect her overall health and beauty. Her hormonal changes can cause the hair to change, generally to a finer, sparser texture. The perspiration from hot flashes can cause the hair to not hold a style very well.

Hot flashes, dizziness, headache, irritability, shortness of breath, disturbed calcium metabolism, and heart palpitations are some of the symptoms. To prevent or help control severe symptoms during "the change of life" the diet should be simple. Eat 60% raw fruits and vegetables, grains, sea food, and protein supplements.

* Avoid dairy products, sugar and meats because these foods cause hot flashes. Include in your diet black strap molasses, broccoli, kelp, dulse, bee pollen, sardines, bananas, avocados, grapes, and beets.

* Avoid meat, coffee, caffeine tea, alcohol, nicotine, and over-processed foods.

* Keep the kidneys clean and give yourself regular enemas or an oral colon cleanser.

* Outdoor exercise, skin brushing, and deep breathing exercise are helpful.

* Your hair style should be low maintenance to allow you to shampoo the hair and scalp frequently to eliminate perspiration. A short natural, braids, twists, and a full hair weave are recommended.

Personalized Hair and Scalp Care....

The overall condition of each person's hair and scalp must be evaluated in order to treat a specific problem. When selecting products for your hair and scalp needs, consult your beautician about your hair type and its condition.

Normal Hair ---is hair that is neither too oily nor too dry. This hair type grows well, has good elasticity, porosity, and has a natural luster and shine.

Dry Hair---is a result of an underactive oil gland that does not secrete enough natural oil onto the hair, causing it to feel hard, brittle, and look dull. (This should not be confused with dry hair due to using the wrong products on the hair.)

Oily Hair---is caused by an overactive oil gland. The gland produces too much sebum for the hair causing it to be heavy , difficult to style, and smelly if not shampooed enough.

Dry scalp---is dehydrated, lacking the natural protective oils that keep it supple. This is recognized by abnormal flaking or dryness that looks as if the scalp is cracking.

Itchy scalp---is caused by oily type dandruff. The skin on the scalp renews itself regularly, pushing old cells off while new cells are being created. However, if these old cells accumulate faster than they are eliminated, this will result in flaking, itchy dandruff.

Once you identify your hair and scalp condition:

1. Select products that will regulate and improve it.

2. Cleanse the scalp of impurities and bacteria.

3. Stimulate the scalp to increase blood flow and to dilate the pores for good penetration of natural oils and treatments.

Healthy hair treatment begins with treating the scalp. Using natural products that prepare the scalp for healing while not adversely affecting the condition of the hair.

Natural Hair Care Recipes...

Scalp Deep Cleanser

1. Mix well 2 egg yolks and 1/4 tsp. of sea salt.
2. Apply to the scalp and massage gently.
3. Rinse with warm water and shampoo with Cornrows & Co. Rosemary Shampoo.

Nutrient Hair Conditioner
1. Shampoo the hair clean.
2. Blend well   2 egg yolks and 2 tbsp. of honey
3. Apply to the hair and leave in for 15 minutes.
4. Rinse with cool water.
5. Style the hair.

Scalp Invigorator
Stimulating antiseptic for the scalp.
Mix 2 tbsp. rosemary oil
    1 tbsp. jojoba oil
    1 tsp white iodine
 Massage into the scalp for 10 minutes, leave in. Do not rinse. Do this twice a week for a tight scalp.

Lemon Rinse
Acid rinse that restores the acid balance, dissolves build-up on the hair shaft, and seals the hair cuticle layer.

1. Shampoo the hair with Rosemary shampoo.
2. Rinse the scalp with a mixture of the juice of 1 lemon & 1 quart of cool distilled water .
3. Apply conditioner rinse to the hair only and rinse after 5 minutes.

Cradle Cap Healer
(for baby)
Apply pure Vitamin E to clean scalp.

Infant scalp care
Mix in baby sink warm water and a little castile soap. With a white, soft wash cloth gently wipe the baby's scalp clean. It is not necessary to shampoo an infants hair the same as you would an adults. Avoid commercial "baby shampoos." They contain fragrance and harsh detergents that can cause irritation.

Natural Scalp Healer
(Excessive dandruff)
Heals irritated scalps and mild seborrheic scaling. Helps to balance the natural acid nature of the skin and hair.
1. Mix 3 ounces of Apple cider vinegar
    1 quart of distilled water
    1 tsp. of sage oil (if available)
Use weekly as the final rinse after a shampoo.   Note:*If the scalp is inflamed and has scabs because of seborrheric dermatitis, consult a dermatologist.*

Cornrows & Co. Hot Oil Treatment
1. Apply Ancient Khemit natural oil formula to scalp and hair.
2. Cover with a plastic cap and use heat cap for 30 minutes (if avail able) or sleep with the plastic cap then shampoo the hair the next morning with Cornrows & Co. Coconut Shampoo.
3. Style the hair in desired design.

13

HAIR CONDITIONERS.......

have become a much needed hair restorer. Although it is believed that hair conditioners repair damaged hair, this is untrue. Conditioners were designed to do what sebum does naturally-- provide a protective coating to the hair, make the scalp and hair supple, and give luster to the hair shaft. With the advent of strong chemical solvents applied to the hair and scalp, the need for hair conditioners is more prevalent.

Cream Rinse Conditioners are finishing agents designed to coat the hair, giving it temporary relief from dryness. The conditioner is applied to the scalp after a shampoo, left on the hair for several minutes and then rinsed off.

Leave-In Conditioner usually has humectants which help to bring moisture to the hair. This type of conditioner is best suited for hair that will be styled naturally or with heat. Avoid using too much leave-in conditioner because it will make the hair sticky, flat, and difficult to style.

Deep Conditioner is a heavier cosmetic such as cholesterol or mayonnaise that is enhanced by heat. (Body heat or electric heat cap). The heat dilates the cuticle imbrication causing the conditioner to penetrate the cuticle layer of the hair shaft.

Hair conditioners are recommended after each shampoo to maintain moisture and give lubrication to the hair shaft. If the hair is extremely damaged, there is not much a hair conditioner can do to restore it. Therefore use the conditioner as a healthy treatment rather than a quick fix measure.

HAIR OIL.......

has been used in Ancient Africa for medicinal purposes. When the scalp does not produce a sufficient amount of sebum on the hair shaft, hair oils can be used to supplement this deficiency. Natural hair oils derived from plants and flowers, occasionally animals (lanolin from sheep oil glands), are used to lubricate, stimulate and keep moisture in the scalp. Avoid heavy synthetic oils (petroleum and mineral oil) that do not absorb into the skin easily creating blockage for the hair follicle and suffocating hair growth.

Some recommended oils:

Jojoba---used by Native Indians. It removes embedded sebum from the hair follicle and makes the scalp less acidic.

Rosemary--- Stimulant

Sage Oil----healer for the skin/scalp

Lemon Oil----has astringent properties

Base oils are used to mix with the above oils:

Olive oil

Almond Oil

Safflower Oil

Castor Oil

It is best to use hair cosmetics that contain these natural oils.

* Massage hair oils into a clean scalp once or twice weekly as needed. Massage in circular motions to help stimulate the blood flow.

* Purchase oils in small quantities so they do not spoil and become rancid.

SHAMPOO........

Shampoos are designed to cleanse the hair and scalp. There is no one shampoo that suits every hair type and hair need. There is no easier method to selecting the right shampoo other than trying several kinds and finding the one that works best for you. There are, however, some basic things that can help you to eliminate certain products based on their specified purpose. For example, shampoo that is designed to make straight hair silky may be too harsh for kinky hair. Kinky hair needs to maintain its natural oils, and shampoos for Caucasian or chemically straightened hair are made to strip the oils from the hair.

Alternate shampoo brands during the year. Your hair condition and hair needs change with the seasons and environment. Therefore, a shampoo that may be perfect in the summer may not be as effective during the winter months. The best shampoo is one that keeps the scalp moist and supple while leaving the hair soft and easy to comb. Look for shampoos that have natural ingredients.

Dandruff shampoos--there are a number of commercial dandruff shampoos that work on mild cases of dandruff. For excessive dandruff accumulation use a shampoo that is gentle enough to use frequently. The common ingredients found in dandruff shampoos are zinc pyrithione, sulfur, and tars which can cause skin irritations or allergic reactions. Use dandruff shampoo in moderation and on the scalp only. To keep the hair from becoming dry use a regular shampoo on the hair shaft.

14

3

The Keys To Natural Hair Care

Pride and Protection

Why I recommend Natural Hair Care

I am a strong advocate of natural (chemical-free) hair care both for its health benefits and its cultural aesthetics. To me, there is nothing more beautiful than a head full of healthy, natural hair. In 1978 I began my hair braiding career from the perspective of an artist. It was my desire to create artistic, African-inspired hair designs.

As braids became the hair fashion, I began to encounter increasing numbers of women whose hair and scalps were extremely damaged. As a means to promote hair growth and self-appreciation to these women that had not experienced healthy hair, my goal then became to re-define standards of health and beauty care. Though I recommend natural styles for black women because they are more becoming than European ones, healthy hair growth has become more important.

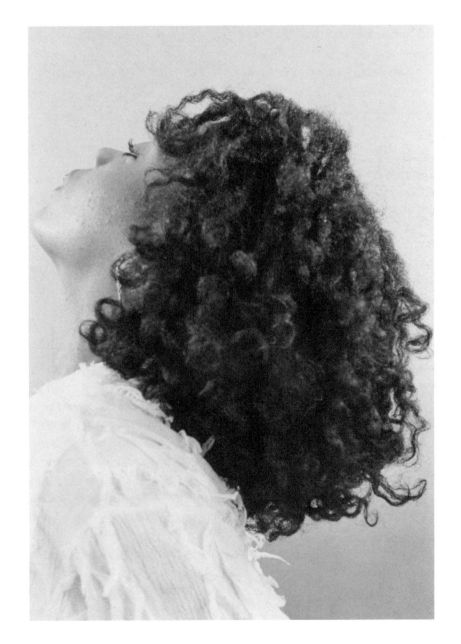

Chemical Hair Abuse

Most of the damage I would see was in some way connected with negligent and/or abusive chemical applications for the purpose of straightening or curly perming the hair. In fact, 95 percent of my clients who had had relaxers or perms had some form of hair damage. And as the years have passed, the hair condition of the general public seems to be getting progressively worse. Today 20 percent of my new clients are permanently bald, in much the same way as male pattern baldness.

It is also a health hazard to the beautician who must inhale the toxic fumes from relaxers, perms, and color products. The FDA has declared that the inhalation of sodium hydroxide causes lung damage. During my training in cosmetology school I had the unhealthy experience of inhaling these toxic fumes for eight hours a day, compounded with aerosol hairsprays and cigarette smoke. I sympathize with beauticians that subject themselves to this for the sake of a dollar and women that suffer great losses for the sake of beauty.

Hair Rehabilitation

Because I braid and style the hair without the use of chemical straighteners or curly perms, I am selected by many women to help them correct their debilitated hair. In other words, because of the dangers of chemical processing, women have begun to realize that professional hair braiding is therapeutically beneficial to their hair. Braids and cornrows are now associated with healthy hair growth. The sad thing, however, is that these women would not come to the salon until their hair was in the worst possible condition.

I am thus challenged to create styles that camouflage damaged hair, while healthy hair grows in its place.

As I stimulate and nurture hair growth for these women, I try to re-educate them on how to take better care of their hair. As a result of this, my role has changed from stylist to hair care specialist, and many of my clients eventually change their negative attitudes towards their natural hair texture. They become proud and protective of their full heads of naturally beautiful hair. They become educated consumers who carefully evaluate their beauticians and the products they apply to their scalps. For this, I hope to gain a generation of educated young women and children who have been taught by their mothers the high value of natural beauty care.

Correcting the Corrective Cosmetologist

I regret to say that the high self- esteem that is instilled by appreciating your natural beauty is not always reinforced by society or the cosmetology industry. Many times African-American women with natural hair styles are ridiculed and questioned by friends and beauticians about their decision not to wear Euro-centric hair dos. In the case of the beautician, this may reflect the industry's desire to sell products and services and their lack of understanding on how to groom our hair. But whatever the reason, it is time that women received some positive, healthy information about the benefits of wearing their natural hair.

Natural hair care is nothing new; it is simply going back to basics and living beautifully like we did in the past. My intentions are to have a positive impact on the young women of today--to offer a holistic, African centered response to the beauty question. In doing so, I hope to correct the "corrective" cosmetology that is jeopardizing the emotional and physical health of African and American women today.

Natural Hair Is Not For Everyone

I have met many African-American women who have expressed deep-seated, negative sentiments about their natural hair. To such women their natural nap is a birth defect. They believe that they are more attractive with European styles and that they can only comb their hair if it is straightened. Their natural hair is not the problem, but their dislike of it is. Unfortunately for them chemically straightening hair care can cause hair and scalp damage, or "transitional" hair breakage. Transitional hair breakage comes from frequently changing styles which change the hair texture. If the hair is over processed, it will eventually break no matter what style they wear. When this occurs, natural hair styles will give the hair the rest and revitalization it needs.

I am frequently asked questions about when, how, and why to "go natural," to grow out all of the chemically treated hair so that virgin hair grows in its place. Although it seems to me that the real question is whether or not it is wise to "go chemical" in the first place, I am offering here a few beauty tips on going natural.

What is Natural Hair?

Virgin hair that is in its original texture and condition as it grows from the follicle is natural hair. The follicle determines the shape and texture of your hair. Hair that has been "permanently" or chemically altered (i.e., by relaxer, permanent waves, curly perms, hair colors) is not natural. Once the hair texture has been chemically altered, it can take up to one year to grow back a full head of natural hair. There are no products, solutions, or procedures that will reverse the condition of chemically treated hair.

Once the hair is relaxed it must grow out and the ends will need to be cut off in order to have natural hair again.

Simply put, natural hair is the hair God blessed you with.

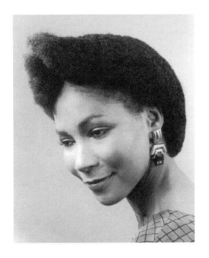

What is natural hair care?

Natural hair care consists of taking care of the hair with naturally derived and wholesome products. It means not chemically altering the hair so that it does not retain its original texture and consistency. It means combing the hair into styles that enhance the natural texture but do not alter the hair strand. For instance, heat pressed or blow-dried hair is still natural, even though heat processes can be damaging to the hair shaft over a long period of time. Braiding, twisting, and styling natural hair are healthy methods that physically change the hair appearance, but do not change the hair texture properties. Choose your braider wisely, however, because incorrect or too-tight braiding can damage the hair and scalp.

Why Should I Go Natural?

Most women decide to wear their hair natural for three reasons: **natural hair care, choice of style, emergency hair therapy, and anchors-a-way.**

Natural Hair care

This woman feels that she is beautiful the way she is naturally. Because she has an honest love of self and appreciation for her hair, she does not feel the need to change, efface or mutilate her hair and beauty with harsh chemicals. To her, natural hair is a part of good living. Because chemicals are known to be unnatural and cause hair and scalp problems, many such women have never chemically styled their hair. They consistently make choices in grooming and styling that are therapeutic, aesthetically ethnic and in accordance with nature and good common sense.

Choice of Style

To this woman, the texture, shape and form of her desired style can only, or best, be achieved with natural hair. Natural hair is her choice mainly for aesthetics. Natural nap gives the snap that holds twisted, locked, braided, and sculptured styles together. Women with naturally or chemically straighten hair often complain that braided styles separate easily and that the styles don't wear as well or as long as they do for women with naturally nappy hair. Many women don't chemically process their hair because it is painful to their scalp and not because they don't like the styles.

Emergency Hair Therapy

I sincerely agree with the old adage "An ounce of prevention is worth a pound of cure." But if and when a woman's hair is balding and badly damaged, hair braiding and natural hair care salons become her emergency room -- or hair trauma unit -- as I sometimes call it. Most women know of the dangers and risks involved in chemically processing their hair, unfortunately they know there are braids and hair extensions available as cover-up solutions so they continue to play Russian roulette with their hair by over-doing chemical and heat processes. In order to give their hair a rest so that it will grow, these women must resort to natural methods of grooming the hair.

Anchors A-Way

Women who wear their hair natural, who have never chemically processed their hair, but use it solely as a means of attaching and anchoring their hair extensions and weave styles. Although they do not like to display their natural hair, they do not want to destroy it for the sake of style. Even though these women do not take pride in their natural hair, they at least value their body enough to protect it. They can now purchase the kind of hair they desire.

Ironically, many of these women will not even let a beautician trim their hair because it is so valuable to them --yet they never show it. Some of these women have had frightening experiences with chemicals in their hair.

Even today many of our elder women wear wigs to cover their natural hair, because they believe this is the acceptable way to wear their hair in public--in the image of the white woman. I remember my great-grandmother wearing a wig to cover her cornrows only when she went downtown and to church. She felt comfortable wearing her simple cornrows at home.

In hair weaves, today's women have found a workable alternative to chemicals. Although wearing a hair weave may hide her natural texture, it is a reasonable alternative to chemically styling the hair.

17

Why Do Women Chemically Straighten Their Hair?

Clients have expressed three reasons why they prefer to straighten their hair:

1. Dislike of kinky, curly hair.

Many women have been socialized to believe that nappy is bad or ugly, and straight is good and beautiful. These women feel more attractive when their hair is straight. They feel they will get better jobs and better men.

One client told me she "would not be caught in public with it unstraightened." She is like many others who are very loyal to their European self-image. Their Colonial upbringing has taught them to hide and deny -- a role of survival in the Western system.

2. Pressure from beauticians.

Some women have confided that they have been ridiculed, badgered and chastised by beauticians for not straightening their hair. One young mother said her beautician called her on the telephone asking permission to give her 10 year-old daughter a relaxer after the mother had emphatically requested a press and curl.

Many cosmetology schools train their students to create styles that can only be done on straight hair texture, so they learn to straighten African-American hair. Consequently, when clients request services other than straightening, many beauticians are at a loss because they are limited in their knowledge and ability to work with natural African-American hair. Such beauticians will, of course, encourage their clients to have their hair permanently straightened in order to make their job easier.

Such beauticians make the argument that hair is difficult to work with if it is not permed. And they claim that to have to press the natural hair only to have it revert back again creates more work for both them and their client. One of my students was told by her cosmetology instructor that her own natural hair was "damaged" because it was kinky. She was told that a relaxer would make her hair softer and healthier. I assured her that African-American women had not been born with "damaged" hair, but that her instructor was a victim of a European-oriented education herself.

3. Fear of messing up or sweating out naturally straightened hair styles. Heat pressing and blow-drying provide a temporary, physical change that is subject to perspiration, shower steam, humidity and precipitation. Even if a woman has a personal distaste for chemical applications, if she prefers straightened smooth Euro-hair styles, she may not want the maintenance hassles of protecting heat-pressed or blow-dried hair styles from the elements. Therefore, she resorts to chemically relaxing her hair.

What does chemical straightening do to the hair?

The chemical used for straightening is sodium hydroxide, which is a caustic soda-lye. (The FDA banned use of more than ten percent of this chemical in household liquid drain cleaners.)[2] If too much alkalis is used, dermatitis of the scalp may occur. Inhalation of this chemical can lead to lung damage.

This chemical works to change the molecular structure of the hair by breaking down the bond. This bond is a polypeptide chain which creates the "S-shaped" kink or curl. Once this bond is broken, the hair loses much of its natural elasticity and resiliency.

The strength (or percentage of chemical) in the relaxer is adjusted for the texture of the hair. Unfortunately, many beauticians think that because hair is nappy, it is coarse in texture. Such a mistaken judgement often causes over-processing.

What about curly perms?

For the permanent curl, thioglycolic acid compounds are used. These thioglycolates are toxic and may cause skin irritation, and absorption into the blood stream may lead to low-blood sugar. Among thioglycolate-related injuries recently reported to the FDA were hair damage, swelling of the legs and feet, eye irritation , rash on ears, neck, scalp and forehead, and swelling of the eyelids. This chemical can also cause severe allergic reactions.[2]

In the process, the hair is in double jeopardy because it is first chemically straightened with sodium hydroxide and then rolled on perm rods, and another chemical (thio) is applied. These chemicals are left on the hair and scalp for a period of time, and then rinsed, and yet another chemical (sodium perborate) is applied to neutralize the acids that curled the hair. Then the client is placed under a hot hair dryer for several hours. Thus, the scalp which has already been traumatized by the chemicals is further distressed by heat.

The greatest danger in using this process is the risk of chemical burn on the scalp which can cause scarring of the tissue. Hair cannot grow through scarred tissue because the follicle holes are closed by the hardened skin. For many of my clients this style has caused permanent hair loss and baldness in the crown of the head.

———————————— 2
A Consumer's Dictionary of Cosmetic Ingredients
By Ruth Winter Crown publisher

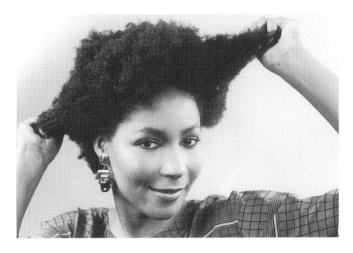

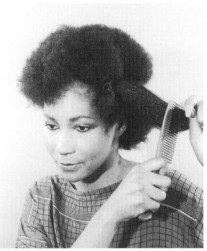

Caring for your natural hair

The beauty of natural hair is that it comes in many textures and curl patterns. Some are large, creating a deep wave in the hair. The opposite end is a small, tight curl pattern, creating a soft, spongy nap. The texture of your hair is determined by your genes and the shape of your hair follicle. The follicle shape for curly, kinky hair is a hole that is curved like a half circle. The follicle for straight hair textures is a straight hole on a slant. Contrary to what cosmetology books and schools teach, African American hair is not difficult to comb, and it does grow considerably long when it is cared for properly. Because this hair type is so unique and varies in texture, the simple *comb-out procedure for natural hair* is all you need to learn in order to prepare your natural hair for styling.

The large round tooth comb, very similar to the combs our ancestors used are best suited for African-American hair. When African women began to comb their hair with the tools and cosmetics designed for European women it was the beginning of a painful, unpleasant experience with our hair. Consequently, "good" hair was believed to be hair "you could get a comb through," and bad hair was believed to break the comb.

Embracing natural hair is the beauty solution for African women . The hair grooming techniques I have developed are simple, easy to do and most importantly healthy for the hair.

21

Shampoo and Comb-Out

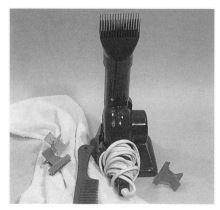

Preparation :

Gather 2 Large towels, *Cornrows & Co. Natural shampoo and hair conditioner*, large tooth comb, butterfly clamps (optional), blow-dryer with a pic comb attachment.

To Shampoo Natural hair:

1. Rinse the hair thoroughly.

2. Apply lathered shampoo to the scalp, hairline, and ends of the hair.

3. Massage the scalp with in and out motions, then stretch the hair to work the lather out to the ends of the hair.

4. Rinse, making sure to remove all of the shampoo. Do a second shampoo then rinse thoroughly.

5. Towel blot the excess water before applying *Cornrows & Co.* hair conditioner; leave the conditioner on the hair for 5 minutes, then rinse thoroughly.

6. Towel blot out the excess water. **(Never shampoo or scrub the hair dry with circular motions. This will ruffle the hair cuticle layer causing the hair to mat.)**

To Comb Out Natural Hair

Start in the front area (on yourself) or the nape area if you are combing out someone else's hair. Part the hair into sections about the size of your palm. The thickness of the hair determines the number of sections. For very thick hair make 10-12 sections, for fine, thin hair make 4-6 sections.

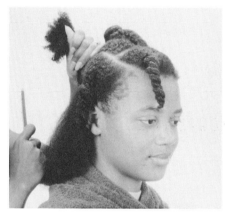

1. Hold the hair firmly close to the scalp with one hand.

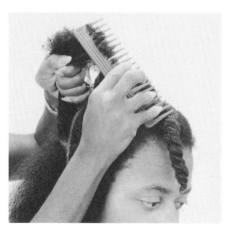

2. Comb-out the ends first, gradually combing down to the hair closest to the scalp. **Comb in gentle plucking movements** and never try to pull through a snarl because this will tighten the tangle.

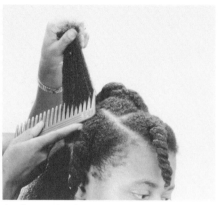

3. Stretch the hair outward as you comb up to the ends.

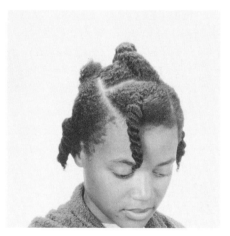

4. After combing out each section, twist the hair loosely to keep it separated. This makes the blow-dry process easier, or you can let the twisted hair air dry naturally for a textured affect.

22

To Blow-Dry Natural Hair

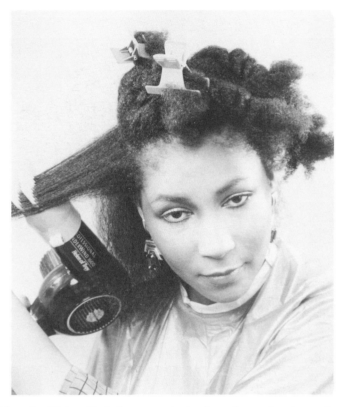

To blow-dry Natural hair the process is simular to the comb-out procedure.
This procedure makes the hair soft and comfortable to comb and style.

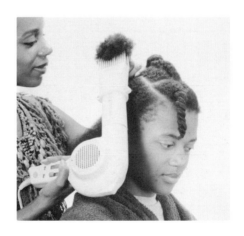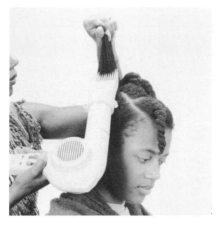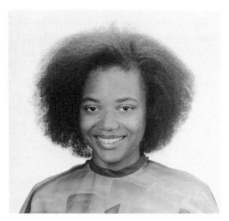

1. Work in small sections, drying the ends first (plucking) at the hair until it is dry and easy to pull the pic through.

2. Gradually work downward to the hair closest to the scalp while stretching the hair outward. This will prevent the hot air from burning the scalp area.

3. After drying each section, the natural hair is ready to be styled.

Five -Minute Natural Hair Styles

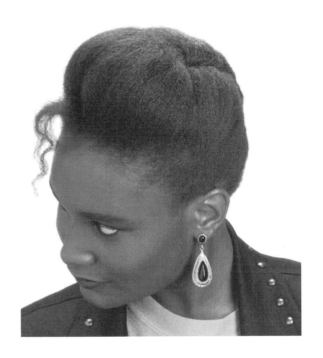

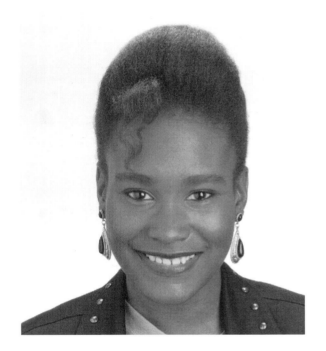

5 - Minute "Beehive Roll"

1. Make a "T" part across the front crown and down the back.

2. At the back center part bobby pin one side flat.

3. With the ends of the other side, fold and roll the hair into the center back, creating a french roll.

4. Fold and roll the ends of the front section to create the front beehive.

5. Curl the front wispy hair.

This classic style works well with natural hair. It is simple and takes only five minutes to do in the morning.

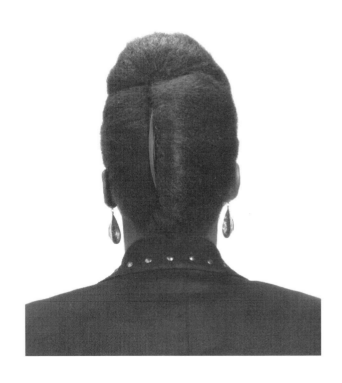

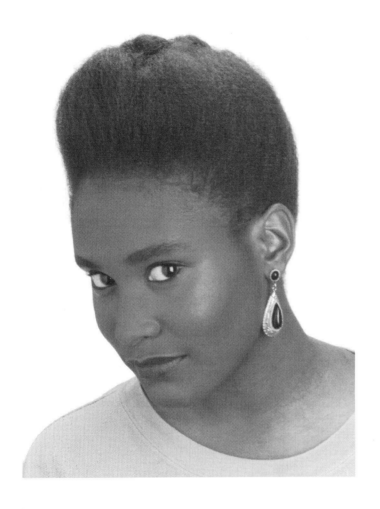

5 - Minute Four Braid Pin-Up

1. Section the hair into four horizontal parts across the head.

2. Loosely braid the ends of each section.

3. Fold and pin each braid to create a row of braids down the back.

4. To smooth the sides and edges, apply a gel and with a scarf tie the hair flat for five minutes.

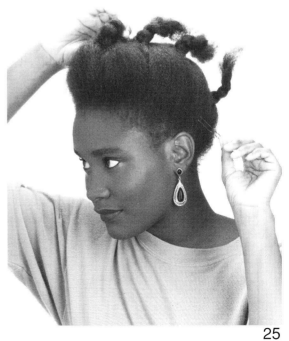

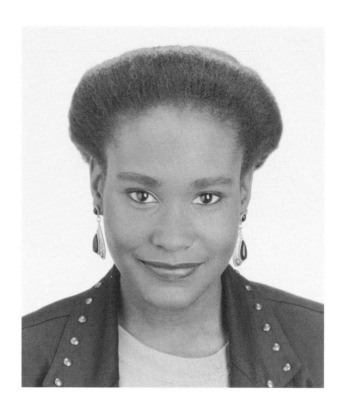

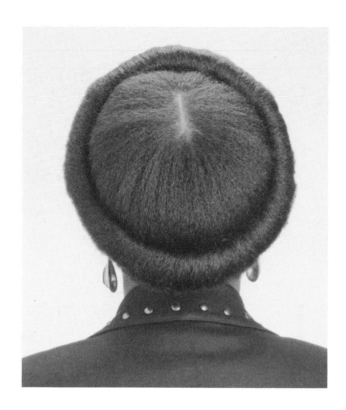

Classic Roll

This no-fuss, no-excuse, natural hair style takes five minutes of your time. It is elegant enough for after-five and a smart look for the working woman.

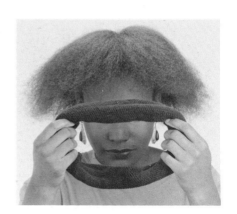

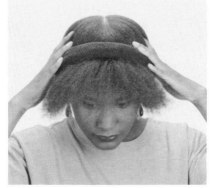

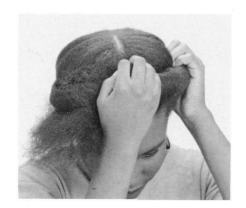

1. Use a tube top or thick head band as the foundation. Comb the hair downward from the center crown.

2. Firmly place the tube top down on the head. Make sure the hair is flat and neatly in place.

3. Tuck and roll the ends of the hair around the tube top.

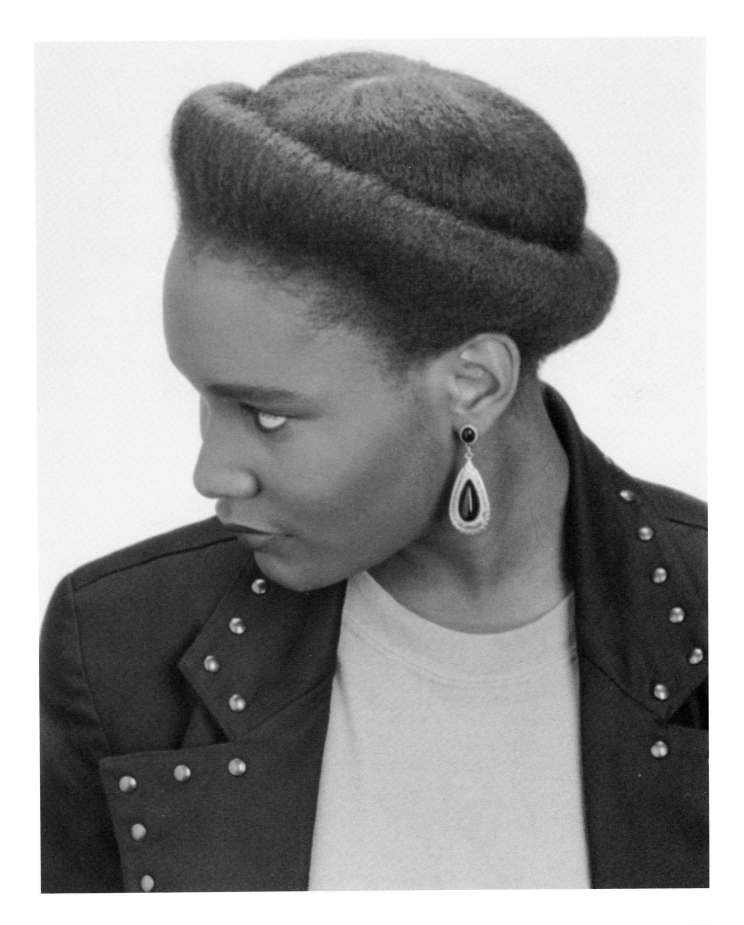

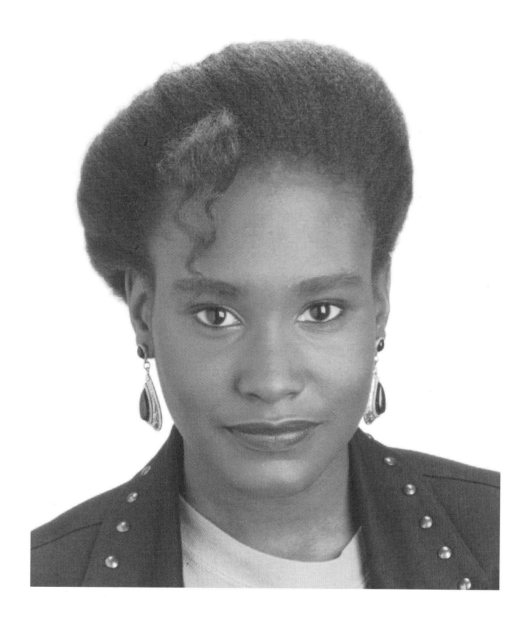

"Variation Of Classic Roll"

This style is created by the same method as the Classic Roll. After rolling the hair around the band, adjust the roll off the face and high on one side.

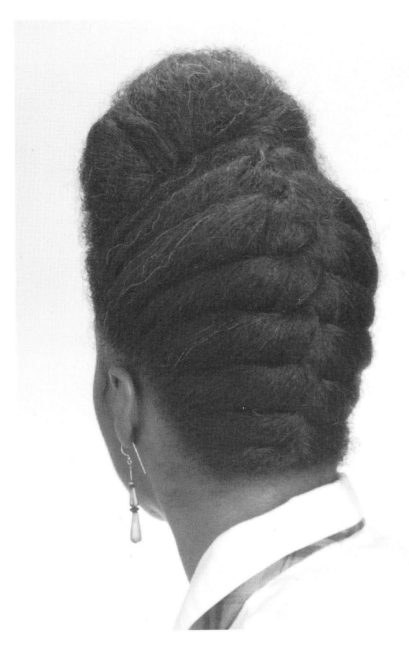

Five minute "African braid"

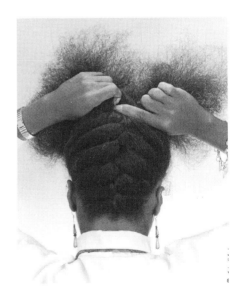

Comb the hair upward, starting at the back neck line, divide the hair into three medium sections. Overhand braid upward and tuck the end into a front beehive roll.

"FLAT TWIST

Flat Twist are soft, versatile, and quick. Perfect style for women on the go, who need to change their style regularly with minimal up keep in between. This style takes an hour to do and will last up to one week.

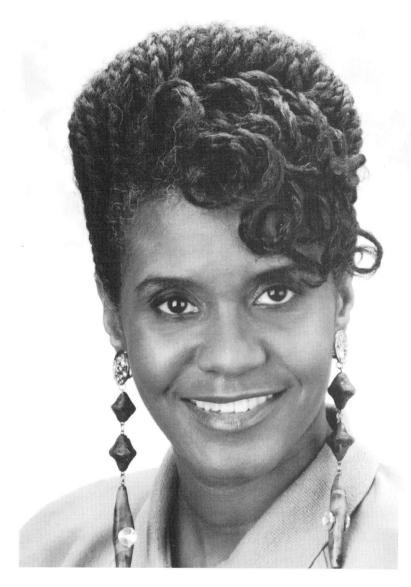

1. Section the hair from ear to ear across the top crown. Flat twist from the nape line up to the part.

2. Individually two-strand twist the front section. Curl the ends of the twist, then fold and roll them to create the crown. Leave free several twist to cascade on the face.

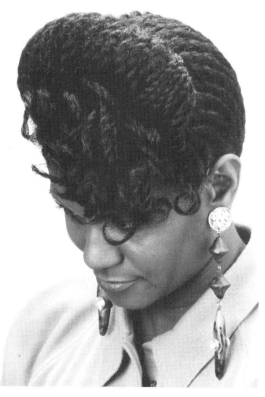

<u>Wear it loose...</u>

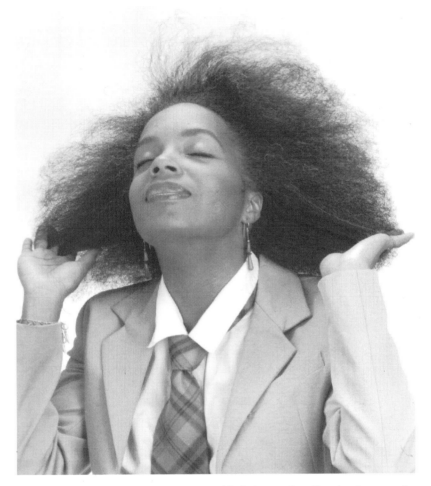

Finger comb and shape your natural hair into a free flowing loose style.
So that the hair looks neat and groomed, keep the ends trimmed regularly.

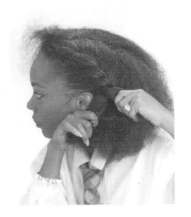

At bedtime make two sections in the hair
and twist or braid the hair on each side.
This will keep the hair loose and textured.

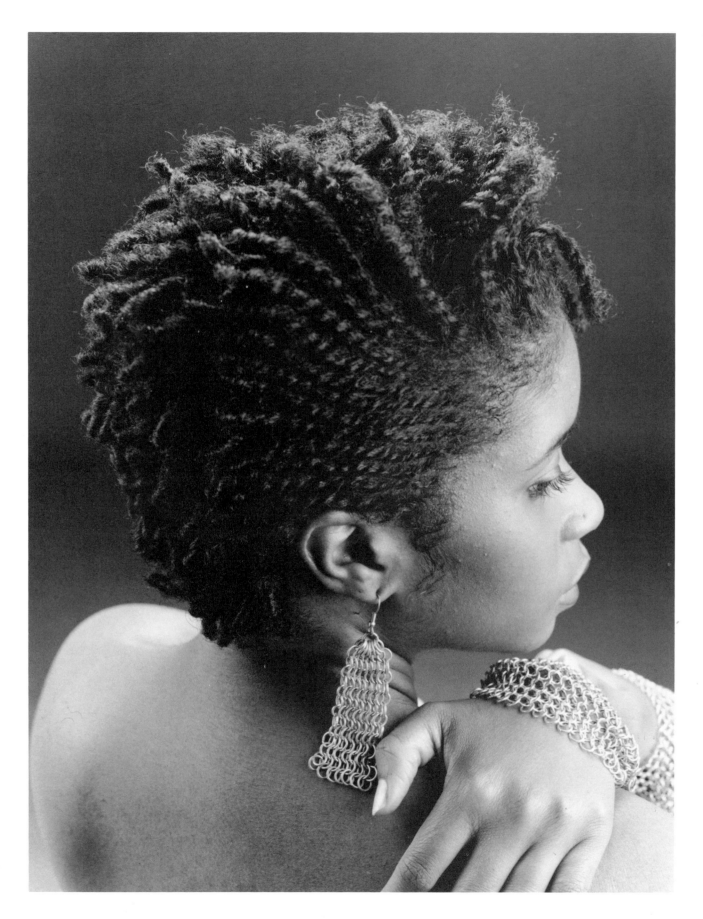

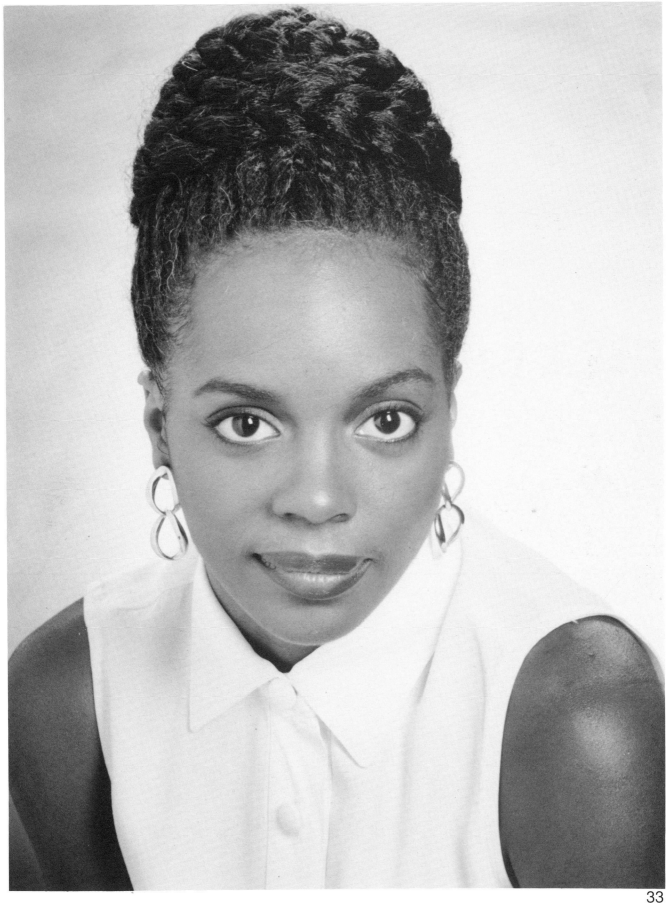

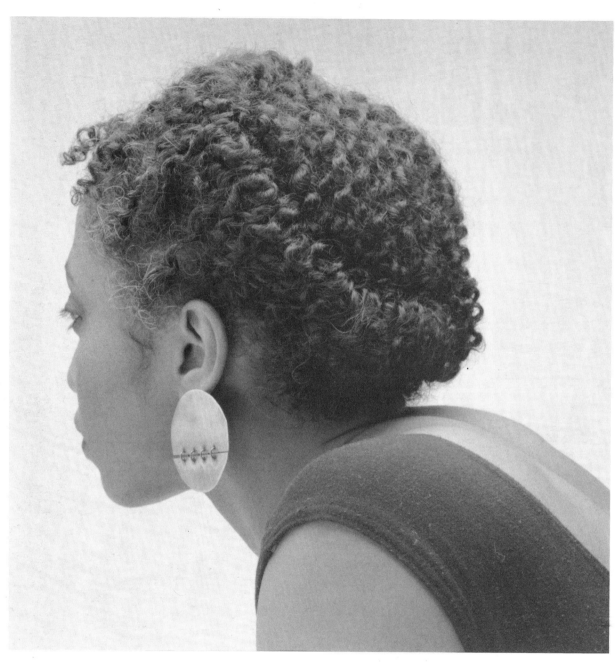

Texturizing with Twist

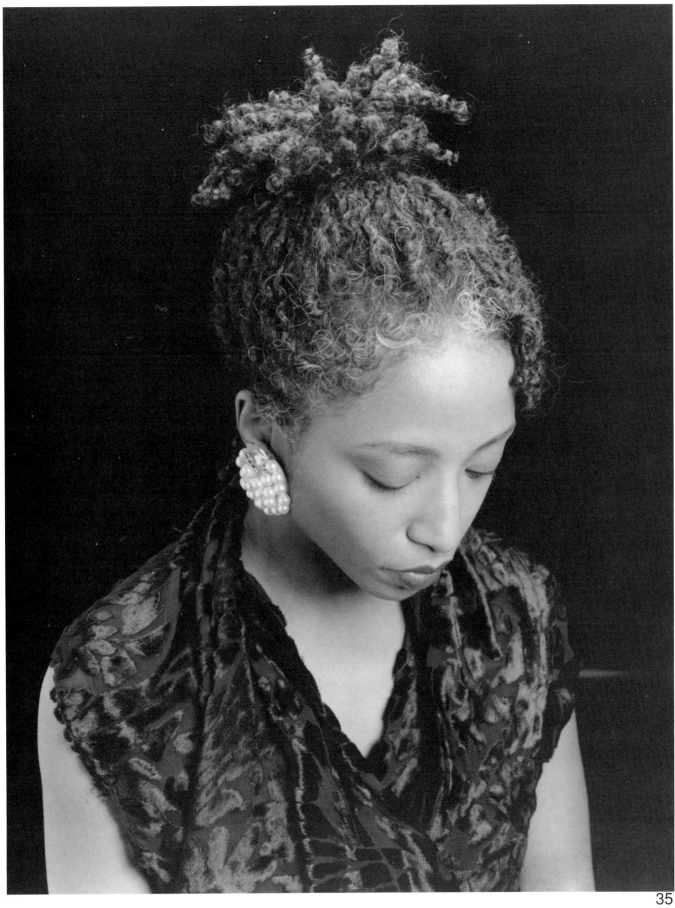

Hair Locks

For many, locking the hair is a part of good living. Hair has a function as far as beauty is concerned. It is our receptor that helps to keep us magnetically balanced. It is the one organ that holds the greatest amount of silicon which is the "feeling" and "magnetic" element of our body. This natural style of unaltered African hair, symbolizes the very Africaness that many have come to misunderstand. The Masai of Kenya, Bushman of Kalahari South Africa, Rastafarian of Jamaica, and African people around the world don heads of natural locks. Because the hair is kept this way for spiritual, cultural, and health reasons: the new resurge of "Black Pride" has made locks a popular style worn by many people for many different reasons. This popularity has created a new service in the hair care industry. Hair stylists are now impelled to open their minds to a natural style that supersedes all previously learned hair styling methods done in the modern salon.

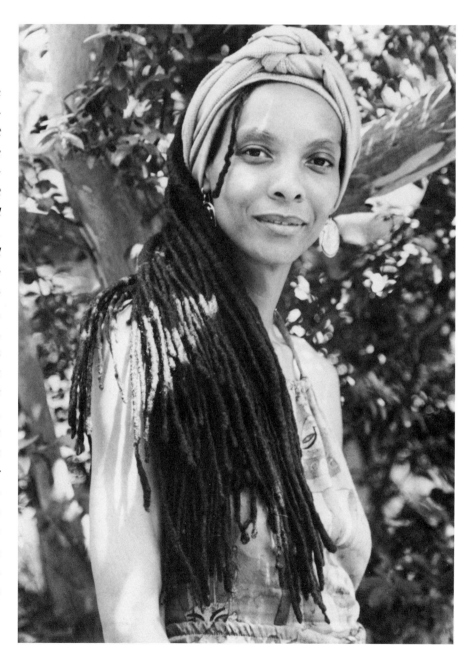

HOW TO GROW LOCKS

Locks can be formed by simply shampooing the hair and allowing it to dry without ever combing or brushing it. This way of locking allows the hair to grow naturally with no uniformity or style design.

"Salon locks" are pre-meditated and trained to grow in a particular shape and size. You or your stylist can start your locks several different ways:

Two-strand twist the natural hair by criss-crossing the hair to form a rope texture. The kink in the hair is what holds the ends together. *(If the hair has been freshly cut, the twist will not hold.)* The twist size will determine the size of the lock. This method gives an almost immediate appearance of locked hair, however, it requires the most grooming.

Individually braid the natural hair in uniform size sections. Shampoo the hair as normal, letting it air dry. Leave the hair braided until the new growth starts to mat and form hair locks. Even though small braids are attractive, if the sections are too small, the locked hair will break off easily at the new growth.

Hand roll small sections of hair between the palms of the hand. This method creates a coiled effect which will eventually begin to lock. To keep the hair from unraveling and frizzing, regular maintenance of re-rolling is needed.

How long does it take the hair to lock?

I have had many clients come to the salon asking for locks as if they can be created in a day. Locking the hair is a process where the hair naturally grows into matted, tangled formations of hair. You cannot make locks with a hair extension or hair cosmetics. The process takes time and patience. If you do not have either, then you don't want locks.

On an average, kinky hair will begin to lock in 4-8 months. Coarser hair will lock faster than soft, curly hair textures. Soft, silky hair can take up to one year to lock. Once this begins, you will need to train and guide the new growth. The new hair will need to be separated and twisted regularly to keep the hair looking neat and fresh.

GROOMING AND LOCK CARE

As the saying goes "Cleanliness is next to Godliness." I cannot emphasize enough the importance of shampooing and grooming the hair. Un-kept, dirty locks give all locks a bad name. Seeing raggedy "dredlocks" perpetuates the idea that people who wear locks do not shampoo their hair. Establish a hair care regiment that allows you the time to regularly shampoo and style your locks. Even though locks require no combing and brushing, well groomed ones require a lot of time and care. "Pretty locks" are regularly shampooed, conditioned, oiled, and retwisted at the new growth.

Tips:

* Shampoo the hair as often as needed. For very thick, long locks allow several hours for the hair to dry completely.

* Shampoo in the shower. Work the shampoo into a rich lather in your hands then massage onto the scalp and hair. Squeeze the lather through the locks to deep clean and remove any lint. Rinse the hair for several minutes to be sure to remove all of the shampoo. To dry the hair, towel blot the excess water squeezing out as much as possible.

* To maintain sheen and luster, apply a light liquid oil throughout the hair.

* During summer months or in hot climate conditions, it is best to let the hair dry naturally. For colder climates, plan to shampoo your hair on a day you do not need to leave the house or dry the hair with an electric dryer.

* Re-twist the new growth every three weeks to keep the new hair looking neat.

* For extremely long locks (seven years and older) if the hair becomes heavy and uncomfortable, cut the ends to eliminate some of the weight.

STYLING YOUR LOCKS

Lock styles are only limited by your imagination. The thinner and longer the locks the more versatility you will have in styling the hair.
Texturizing...Dampen the hair first, then depending on the desired effect use one or more of these texturizing methods. (Criss-cross twist several locks together, braid the locks into sections, roll the locks on sponge or perm rod rollers or wind the locks into a pin curl.) Let the hair dry completely. Once the hair is dry untwist, unbraid, or unroll the locks. These different texturizing methods create different styles. The twist and braids will give the locks a wavy affect. Rollers create a curly full body style.
Coiffed Locks.... Locks that are pliable can be manipulated into shapes, forms, and many hair designs. For the office you can style the locks into contemporary rolls, beehives, and chignons. And for a dramatic look, cut the locks into a precision style.

"God answered my prayer, for one night I had a dream and in that dream a big black man appeared to me and told me what to mix up for my hair. Some of the remedy was grown in Africa, but I sent for it, mixed it, put it on my scalp, and in a few weeks my hair was coming in faster than it had ever fallen out. I tried it on my friends; it helped them. I made up my mind I would begin to sell it."
Madam C.J. Walker, 1905

Madam C.J. Walker started a cosmetics manufacturing company in 1910, providing job opportunites for black women while training them her system for healthy hair care. To bolster the confidence and self-esteem for black women during a time when they did not feel valued in American society, she encouraged her agents to open their own businesses, contribute part of their earning to charities, and to take great pride in their personal appearance and to give their hair proper attention.

A'lelia Perry Bundles; Madam C.J. Walker entrepreneur Chelsea House Publishers, New York Philadelphia

4

Female Hair Loss and Balding

BALDING AND HAIR LOSS

Hair shedding, thinning, falling, and receding all translate into balding. Although the actual cause of hair loss and baldness is unknown, scientific research has shown that in many cases there is an impairment of the blood supply to the hair root. I believe, however, that while some hair loss is inevitable in these modern times, knowledge of ways to stimulate healthy hair growth and prevent premature hair falling can assure that women will have a healthy head of hair all of their lives.

There are many factors that affect hair growth and accelerate hair loss. Hair loss can be directly attributed to abusive hair care, poor diet, vitamin deficiency, stress, and iron deficiency. Pregnancy, acute illness, HIV , poor circulation, thyroid disorder, chemotherapy, drugs, radiation, diabetes, hormone imbalance, lupus, and age can indirectly cause hair to thin and bald. Whether you are losing your hair because of heredity, illness, or abuse, understanding what stimulates the blood circulation will be of great benefit in affecting your hair growth.

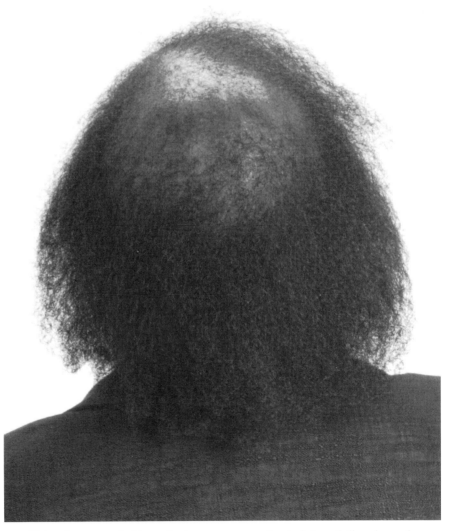

(Fe)male pattern baldness in the crown area, due to internal disorder and external trauma to the scalp.

Hair Growth Cycle

Hair growth is determined by your genes and hair type. The average person grows 1/2 inch of hair per month or 6-7 inches per year. Because women are constantly cutting, burning, or damaging the hair shaft as fast as it grows, they do not experience their normal hair growth cycle. Many negligent hair care practices have stunted the growth process for years.

Depending on the texture and area of the head, hair tends to grow faster in certain places. Soft fine hairs along the hairline grow slower than the hair in the crown of the head. Therefore it is a good practice to handle the soft hair with care so that you do not damage it. The natural process of the growth cycle is for old hair to shed, and new hair to replace it. It is normal to shed of 50-100 strands per day if it is replaced by the same amount. Most shedding generally happens in the morning. If the hair is shedding in excessive amounts and not replacing itself at the same rate, this can lead to hair loss and baldness.

Hair Abuse

Women sacrificing healthy hair for the sake of style is probably the most common reason for hair loss. Often these women treat their hair as if it were made of steel. This attitude usually starts during childhood where traction alopecia -- hair loss due to extreme tension and pulling on the hair -- is found on young girls whose parents placed too tight braids, rubber bands, or barrett's in their hair. The tension causes pustules (small white pimples) along the hairline that can become infected leading to permanent hair loss. Because of this malady, many young African and American girls are bald along the hairline before they reach adolescence.

On my visits to West Africa, it was common to see young girls and women with a two-inch bald hairline. This type of hair loss can be easily prevented and is only "hereditary" by the fact that parents commit the same mistakes generation after generation.

Another form of hair abuse is the foolish notion that possessing a straight, sleek hairline is more important than the hair itself. Daily pressing of the soft curly, kinky, hairline will more than guarantee hair loss. If the follicle has not been damaged, stopping the daily hot combing will allow the broken hairline to grow back.

Right here, let me say emphatically that it is not normal for women to lose their hair the way many men do. In my thirteen years as a hair care specialist, I have seen an alarming increase in the numbers of women who have a hair loss problem that closely resembles male pattern balding. The two things these women had in common are that they were all between the ages of 30-50 and all had worn the "curly" perm for some period in their lives.

Women today should know that it is a fact that the prolonged use of relaxer and curly perms can cause hardened scalp tissue and hair loss. Scarred scalp tissue can block the hair follicle. A Swedish scientist, Lars Engstrand, M.D. presented conclusive evidence that baldness in men is caused by pressure on the capillaries of the scalp by a thickened tendinous membrane (galae) located on the top of the head.[3]/ In women, this membrane remains thin and elastic throughout her life. Therefore, it is certainly not normal for women to bald like their fathers.

The result of this new type of baldness in women where the production of new hair has ceased can be related to one or more of the following: obstruction of the blood circulation to the hair follicle and/or hormonally influenced obstruction of circulation to the scalp in the case of women during the Summer and Autumn phase (menopause, hysterectomy).

For Spring and early Summer women, who should still have full heads of hair, I cannot stress enough the dangers related to prolonged chemical hair treatments.

However, if you are currently suffering from the type of baldness described here, there are natural hair care remedies and styles to prevent further hair loss and to alleviate embarrassment from this condition. Extreme hair loss in the crown area can be safely covered by a full hair weave.

Medical Causes of Hair Loss

Thyroid and pituitary gland disorders can cause hair growth problems. The pituitary gland distributes hormones to other parts of the body. The over or under production of hormones certainly affect hair growth. Under these circumstances a woman needs a healthy diet and the care of a physician.

Hair lost because of pregnancy, hormonal imbalance, illness and medical treatments will usually grow back when the condition is healed. Many of my clients who were receiving chemotherapy treatments experienced hair thinning and texture changes in their hair. Hair becomes very soft and fine during these treatments.

Most clients wore a wig during this time to cover the hair loss so not to cause styling stress on their fragile hair. I would give these women moral support, and realistic hair care options until their hair eventually grew back. Today all of these women have thick, normal hair growth. And in some instances their hair is even stronger than before.

---
[3]
Stop Hair Loss, by Dr. Paavo Airola, Health plus publishers

Natural Hair Changes

As women age, their metabolism will naturally slow down. Hormone changes during the "change of life" will cause hair to thin and not reproduce as quickly. There is not a lot we can do to stop the graces of age. However, we can maintain a healthy head of hair if we exercise, eat well, and use sound hair care regiments in the younger years.

Alopecia Areata

Premature hair loss that appears in small round areas about the size of a silver dollar is caused by internal disorder or disease that has affected the nervous and/or immune systems. Such diseases may be syphilis, nervous disorders, anemia, and typhoid fever. Scalp massage, scalp stimulation, cleansing diet and treatments have proved very helpful in alleviating this condition.

It won't grow anyway

Despite all the hair loss problems that women experience, many cases could be prevented if they simply change their ways. Women suffering from illness and early signs of hair thinning who continue to put lye and other caustic products on their already fragile hair are asking for further troubles. The defeating attitude, "It doesn't matter what I do to it, it won't grow anyway," is the worst culprit and perfect excuse for women to abuse their hair.

A client's mother came to my salon after years of struggling to get her hair to grow. This late Autumn woman was bald around the hairline and had straggly thin hair ends from an over-processed curl she had been wearing

for years. She had always trusted her beautician to take care of her hair, believing that her hair loss problems were a result of "bad hair" and not because of excessive chemical treatments. This woman's hair was naturally fine and delicate, and required only basic hair care. Her fine hair was literally being dissolved by the harsh chemicals, and this had impeded its growth over the years.

Today, her hair is silvery gray, healthy and growing below her shoulders.

Through natural hair care, many of my clients have discovered their maximum hair growth potential, and they have learned to maintain a healthy head of hair. The points that I want to make here are : (1) that African-American hair will grow if taken proper care of and (2) that it is never too late to care for your hair, if you are willing to appreciate it and work with its natural texture.

EXTERNAL STIMULATION TO PROMOTE HAIR GROWTH

Now that you understand the importance of a healthy diet and mental attitude, here are some tips on how to encourage blood circulation to the scalp through external stimulation.

Daily Brushing ----

Always use a natural bristle brush. Hair brushing loosens dirt and debris from the hair shaft. It stimulates blood circulation and lifts dead skin cells, opening the pores to release toxins from the skin.

Scalp Massage ----

An often overlooked remedy that revives hair immediately. Do this in the privacy of your home using your hands or a vibrating massage machine.

Not only does this encourage blood circulation, but it rejuvenates and energizes the whole body.

Upside-Down Hair Care---

This Ancient Indian Yoga technique sends blood rushing to the scalp and hair follicle. When relaxing at home, elevate your feet or stand on your head for 10 minutes daily. Another way to increase circulation to the tiny blood capillaries in the scalp is to lie on a slant board which is raised about 20 inches on one end. You can make this yourself with a solid board propped against the bed or propped on a 20" wood block.

MALE HAIR LOSS

Male pattern balding is a hereditary trait that affects some men. The cause and cure are unknown. However, there has been much research to suggest that the hair condition due to hormonal stimulation and the amount of blood which each male has available to the scalp is influenced again by a hereditary trait. Some experts have suggested that beginning at age 18 the tendinous membrane located in the crown of the head becomes thick and hardened in some men. This thickened membrane then creates pressure and tension on the scalp which causes impaired blood circulation and nourishment to the hair papilla. The gradual decrease in the hair growth and the ability to reproduce hair in this area results in baldness.

A beautiful bald head is therefore inevitable for some men, but with proper early hair care education, the onset of this condition can be prolonged.

If there are bald men in the family on the mother or fathers side, the likelihood is that he to will probably experience this family trait.

HIS LEARNING HAIR CARE.....

The sensual act of touching is usually taught by the female (mother) to her male child. Because it is the mother's touch that he experiences first it is natural and healthy for a male to touch her back. I often assure my clients that it is okay for her male child to comb the dolls' hair and even to comb her hair. This is an act of loving, nurturing, and caring. If the male learns this at and early age, it will not seem "girlish" to pamper and take time to care for himself or his daughters' hair. I've heard men say they "don't use shampoos and conditioners because all that is not necessary for men." Many male hair problems are caused by the inferior products they use. Some of our great hair stylists are men, and some of our most caring hair dressers have been our dads. Fathers have braided, combed and tried to do the best they can taking care of their daughters hair.

When I produced "Thunder Head Hair Care Video for Moms & Dads," I was impelled by fathers who would seek answers to the most basic questions about hair care for their daughters. These fathers are very proud and concerned that their daughters' hair is combed pretty. As a result of not learning how to shampoo, comb out, blow dry, and braid hair, the responsibility would be frustrating for fathers and painful to the child. With the help of the hair care video, men can now take some responsibility in healthy hair care for themselves and their children.

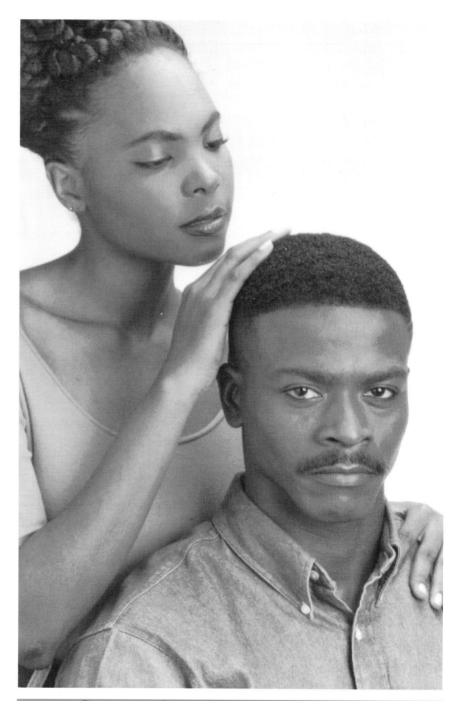

Caring for your man's hair...

42

TIPS FOR MALE HAIR CARE

For your man doesn't quite know what to do about his hair care...

1. Help him select the types of products that are good for his hair texture (i.e shampoo, conditioner, combs, brushes).

2. Show him how to use the products correctly so he does not use a bottle of shampoo a week. Men can shampoo their hair twice a week using a very small amount of shampoo. Too much shampoo will cause the hair to look dull from a film build-up .

3. He should not shampoo the hair with soap. This will make the hair dry, coarse, and ashy looking.

4. Give your man a scalp massage at least twice a month. Apply a natural oil (jojoba, olive, safflower, or castor oil) to the scalp. Massage in circular motions for 10 minutes. Shampoo and rinse the hair.

5. Do not use chemicals (perm, relaxer or the curl) to soften the hair. A good haircut makes the hair soft and easy to comb through. Straightened hair for men is feminine, unhealthy, and quite vain.

6. For fine or naturally straight hair textures try a scissor haircut so that the hair does not stick out.

7. If he has male pattern baldness, he should have his barber/stylist keep the hair around the edges cut very short and close. Short hair detracts from the bald area. Long hair around a bald area makes the bald spot appear larger.

8. Daily hair brushing is important for men. This will stimulate the blood circulation and encourage the natural activity of the oil glands. The natural oils will give the hair natural sheen and luster.

Natural hair care remedies for male balding

1. Rub aloe vera gel into the scalp daily at a young age.

2. Weekly strong herbal hair rinse of nettle, rosemary, and sage.

3. **Grandpa's Shotgun Hair Concoction.**
Mix :
   Fifth of vodka
   1/3 cup of cayenne (red) pepper Let this mixture sit for 10 days. Strain the pepper and rub small amounts of the concoction onto the crown area of the head twice a week. (*This mixture helps to revitalize the scalp, stimulating blood circulation, and dilating the pores to prepare the the scalp for other treatments.*)

43

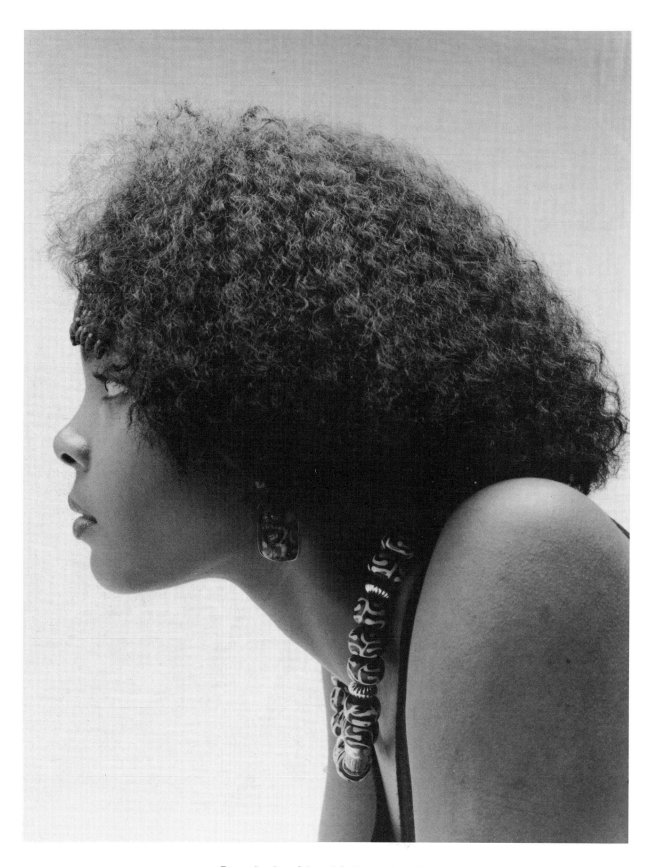

Interlock with a kinky extension.

44

5 Hair Extensions

Hair extensions are beauty ideas which originated in Ancient Africa where Nubian and Egyptian women wore many styles of wigs made from natural hair, plant fiber, and wool. These intricately designed head coverings protected them from the hot sun's rays and were worn for social festivities and ceremonial rituals. Ancient warrior queens, such as Hatshepsut, Cleopatra, and the Queen of Sheba wore military wigs that were braided short and helmet-like. African women often shaved their natural hair close and wore wigs for religious, social, and hygienic reasons.

Because of the variety of colors and textures available, hair extensions can be worn by women of any age, race, or socio-economic status. Although I recommend simple cornrows with no extensions for children, if the hair is thin, short or damaged, minimal hair extensions can be worn even by the young (older than five years old).

Many women wear hair extensions solely for style , but women suffering with problem hair have found them beneficial as a cover and protector for their recuperating hair. The entertainment industry with its emphasis on maximum beauty has made hair extensions a very popular style alternative.

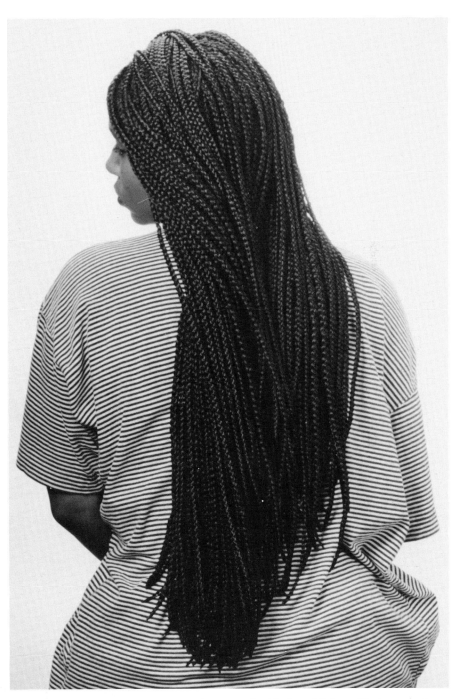

Braids, twists, and cornrows can be created with the addition of hair extensions. *Hair extensions are added to many contemporary braid styles to give fullness, length, and longevity.*

45

Modern techniques of hair extensions

Today hair extensions still serve as adornment for social, therapeutic and protective purposes. Although, the adding of synthetic or natural hair can be achieved by several methods, a braid foundation has proven to be the safest and most versatile of all hair addition techniques. Hair weaving, interlock braiding, lace braids, thread wrapping, cornrows, and individual braids are some of the recommended hair extension techniques. Other methods, such as bonding, glue, and fusion, were developed as a result of the braid techniques. However, these methods are messy, unsafe, and can be damaging to the hair shaft. Good common sense suggests not to put glue-adhesive on the hair. It does not wash out easily and will rip the hair where it is applied. Equally as damaging are braid methods performed by unskilled persons.

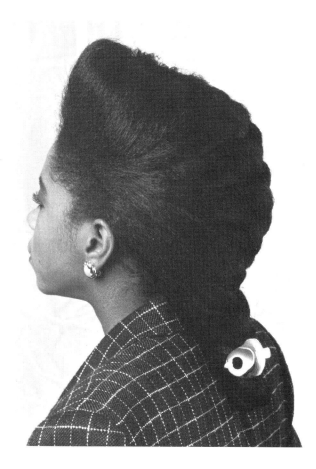

Various methods of hair extensions include:

Hairweaving--- is accomplished by first cornrowing the natural hair in horizontal or circular patterns called tracks. Then wefted rows of hair extension are sewn onto the tracks.

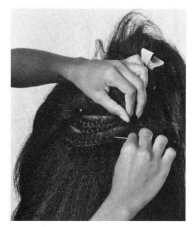

This method is quick and adds no stress to the natural hair.

The advantage of a full hair weave is that all of the natural hair is covered by the extension, thereby allowing a change of hair color, texture and length (shorter or longer) without the use of chemicals.

The disadvantages of hair weaving are that it can be costly to maintain, and it is difficult to conceal the tracks in extremely windy weather (nothing a hat or scarf cannot resolve). This method works well for all women, but it is especially well suited for women in the Summer and Autumn phases who are experiencing noticeable hair thinning. It is also recommended for women who have damaged hair that needs a "hair rest." This style of extension will give you the therapeutic benefit of braids without actually seeing the braids.

You should allow at least two hours to have this style performed by an experienced professional.

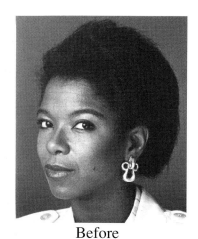

Before

Five tracks of synthetic extension were added to this client's 3" length hair.

46

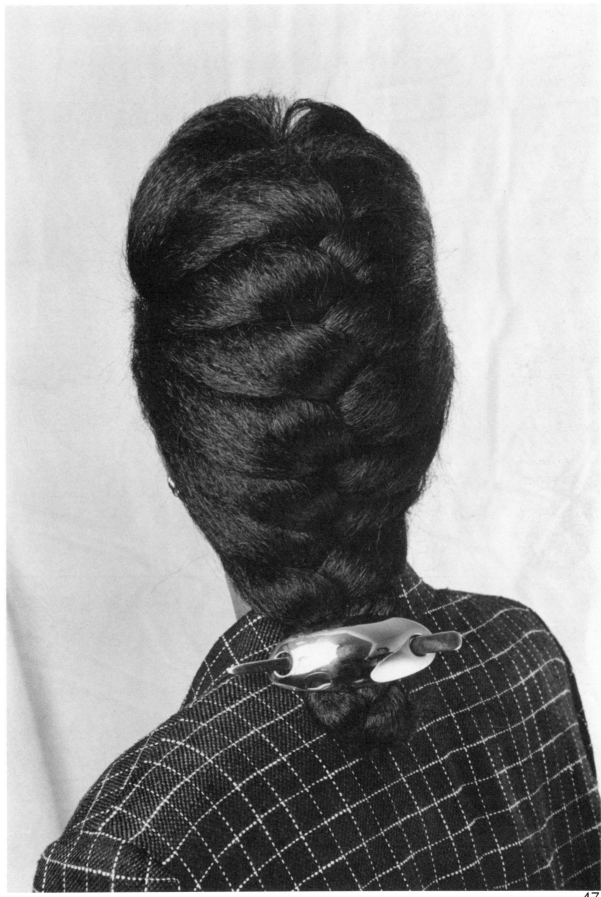

Interlock-Braid is a cornrow method where very small amounts of extension are added to each stitch of the braid. The finished look shows only the added loose hair extension. This style gives a very natural flow to the extended hair.

The disadvantage of interlock braids is that straight texture hair extensions loosen quickly and may expose the cornrows at the crown of the head. This method can take up to three hours to complete and will last for six weeks.

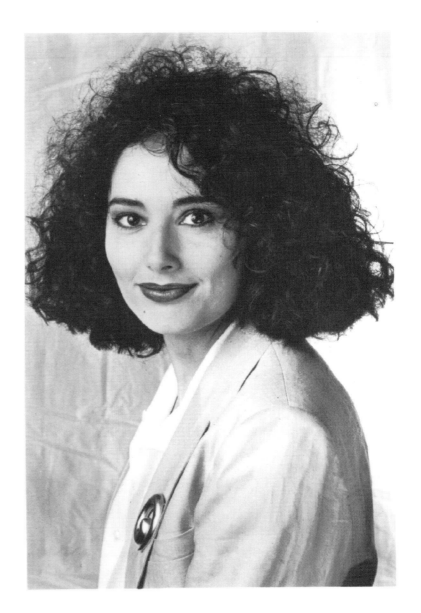

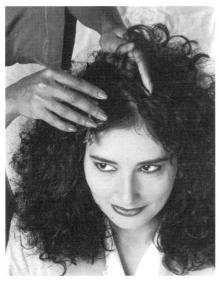

Without using chemicals we are able to give this client a curly perm style, using cornalon fiber and the interlock method.

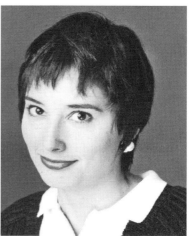

BEFORE

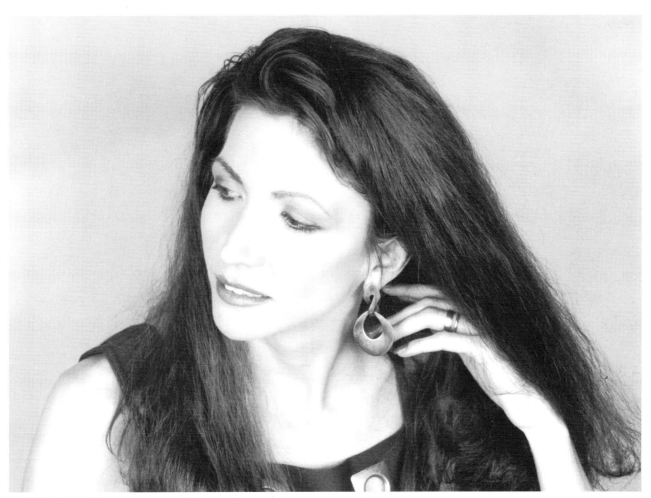

This client did not want to wait for her layered cut to grow out to one length. Five rows of Cornalon weave extension was added to attain an instant long hair style.

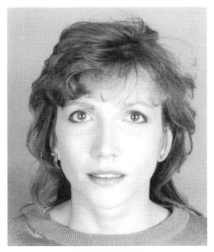

BEFORE

To change the style to an elegant updo, pin the back into a french roll and curl the front.

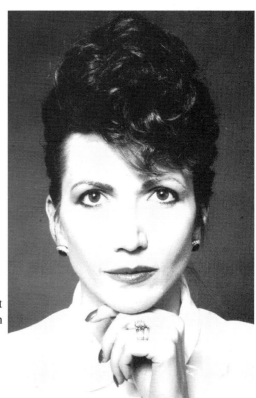

49

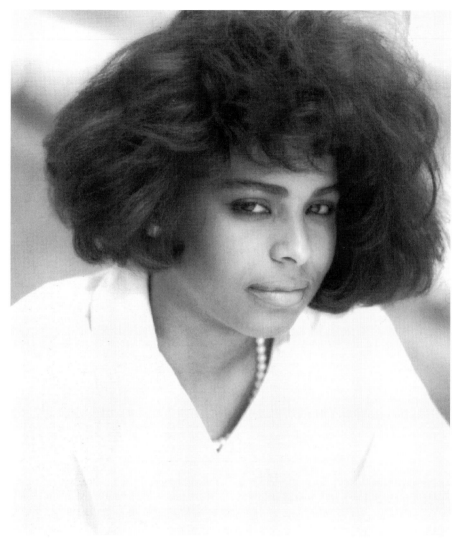

__Full hair weave design to cover this clients natural hair__

ends of the hair extension. Rinse the hair thoroughly under a gentle shower. Depending on the type of hair extension, select a conditioner that is suited for its texture. To dry the hair wait thirty minutes for the hair to partially air dry then blow dry and style as you desire. If your textured extension is krimpy, curly or wavy allow the hair to air dry completely to maintain the texture.

THE DIFFERENCE BETWEEN HUMAN AND SYNTHETIC HAIR EXTENSIONS?

Human Hair Extensions-- offer great styling versatility like the natural hair. This extension can be colored and texturized to match most hair types.

The disadvantages are availability, cost and quality. Human hair extensions are usually more expensive, and prices will fluctuate depending on supply and demand. The availability of good quality human hair extensions can be limited, and if the quality is poor, the hair will surely matt, tangle, look dry and not style easily.

Synthetic Fiber Extension--- is a man-made material designed to resemble hair. Most fiber extension is made from a plastic resin, or a modacrylic fiber. Synthetic hair as it is generally referred to is durable, widely available and best-suited for certain hair styles and hair textures. In addition to being considerably less expensive than human hair, advanced technology has produced synthetic fiber extensions in a wide array of natural looking colors and hair textures. The Cornalon hair extension is a specially designed fiber that closely resembles "real" hair.

EXTENSION WEAR?

Most extension styles will last up to two months. Soft, fine, and straight hair textures may loosen faster than curly, coarse hair. After two months of wear the hair extension should be remove so that the new grown hair can be combed out thoroughly to prevent it from tangling and matting to the extension. Avoid wearing the same extension for extremely long periods, this can cause hair and scalp problems.

SHAMPOO AND CARE FOR EXTENSIONS

Extensions should be considered a part of your natural hair when shampooing and grooming. Shampoo and condition the hair no more than once a week with the best products available. For at home care, it is best to shampoo the hair in the shower, rinsing thoroughly, work the shampoo into a thick lather and massage gently in between the braids on the scalp. Gradually work the lathered shampoo through to the

50

Remember these tips:

* Avoid using oils, gels and hair sprays on human hair extensions. Such products cause residue build-up making it difficult to style.

* Synthetic extensions are recommended for swimming since the texture does not change when it is wet.

* Synthetic extensions can be permanently curled into various configurations.

* Do not relax your hair before adding extensions or after the extensions are applied; chemicals weaken the hair condition making it prone to breakage.

* Consult with your professional braider about your hair extension maintenance.

* Avoid using products that contain alcohol because this will have a drying affect on the hair.

* When shampooing the hair never scrub in a circular motion, this will ruffle the hair cuticle and cause it to tangle.

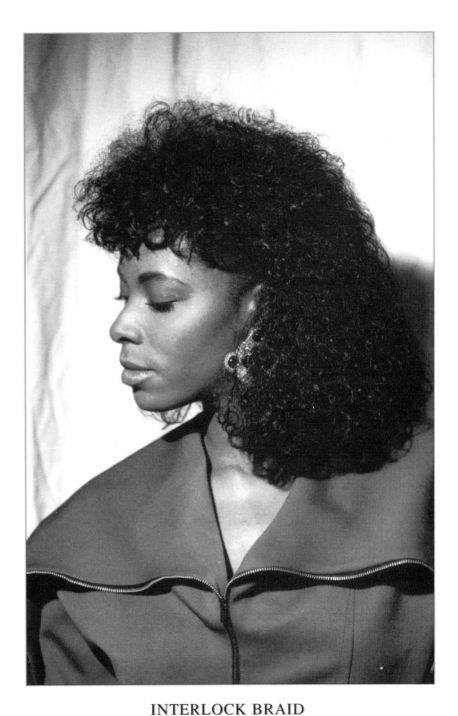

INTERLOCK BRAID

A combination lace and interlock method was used to create this style.

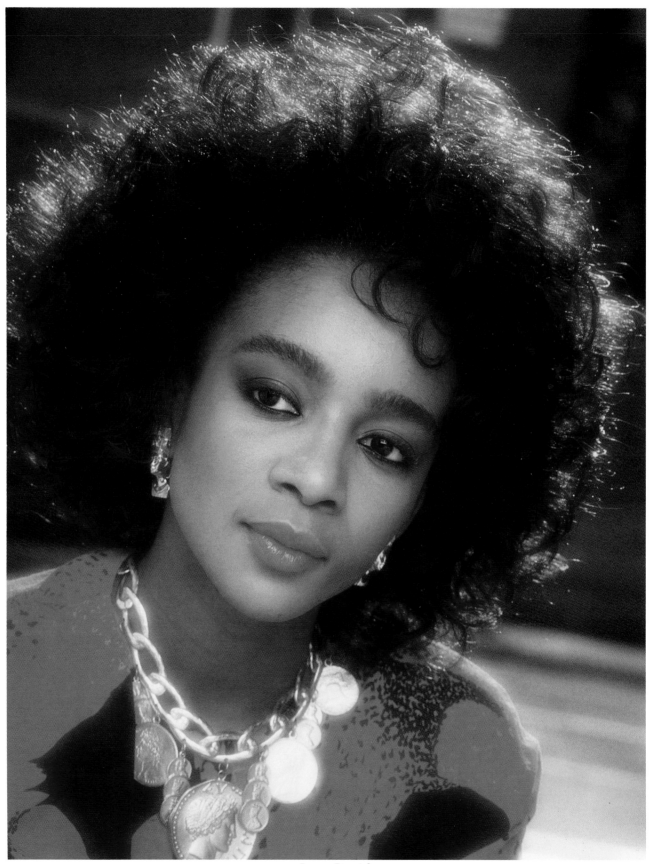

Lace Braids

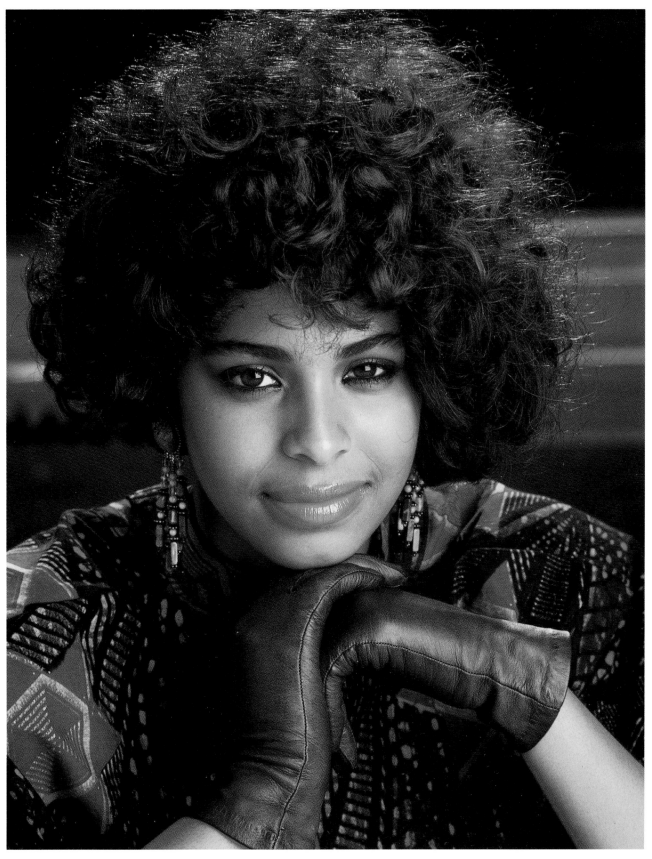

Hair Weave

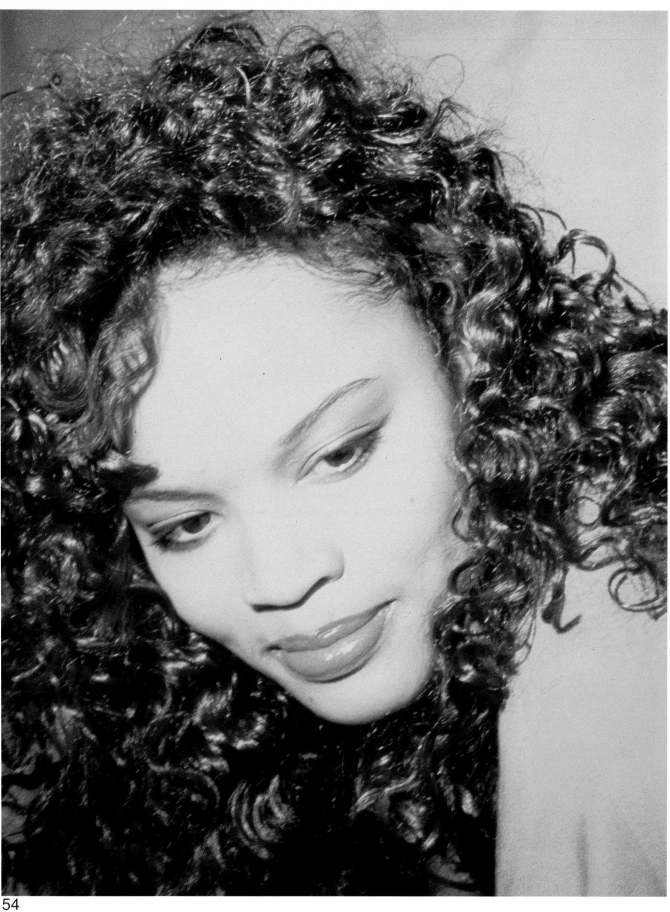

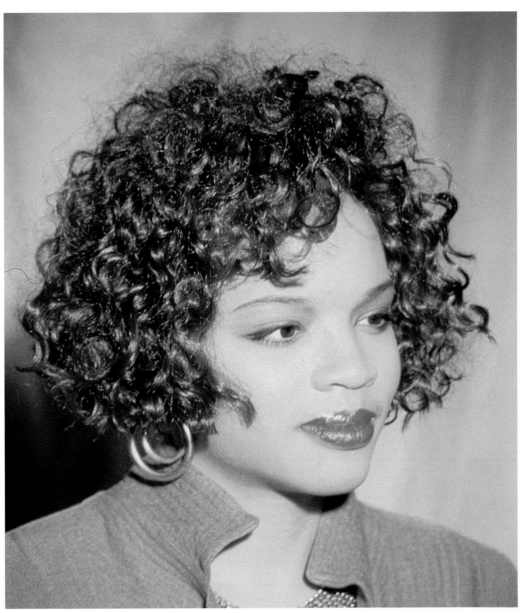

A curly cornalon extension was added to cover all of this clients hair. While giving her chemically treated hair a rest, she can enjoy the freedom of textured hair extensions.

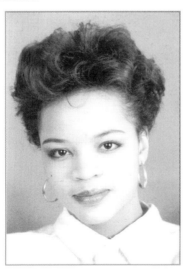

Before

LACE BRAIDS

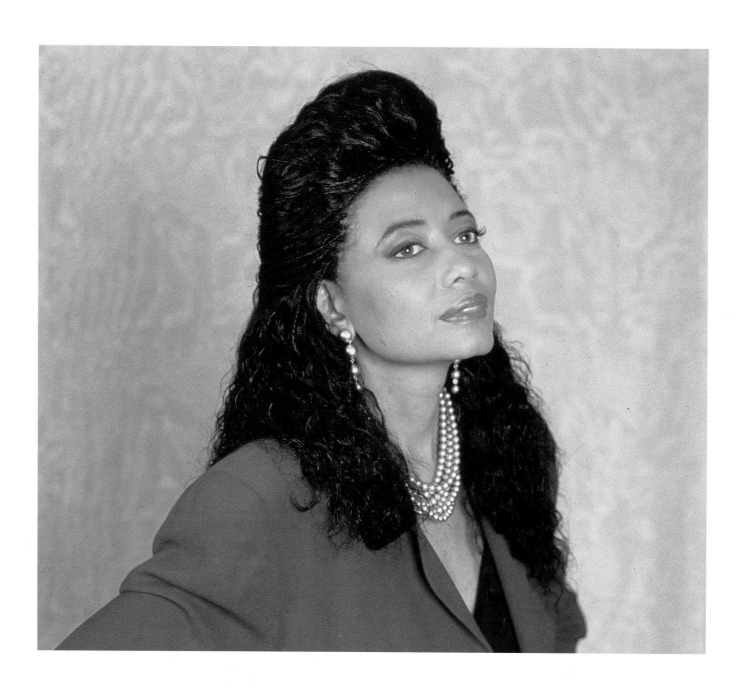

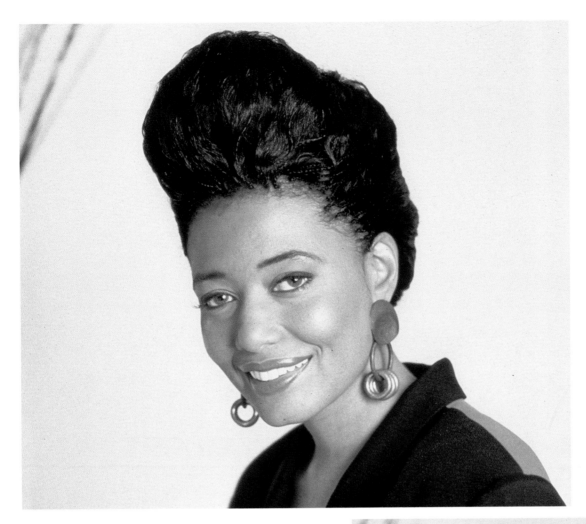

Lace Braids-- are the same technique as individual braids, except that a small piece of the hair extension is left out at the begining to cover the entire braid.

Unlike the interlock braid method the lace braid style cannot be cut shorter than the natural hair length because the extension is braided down to the length of the natural hair. Even though this style is designed to cover most braids, in some instances they may show through. This is a great style for women who want extensions with versatility. This method takes at least eight hours to do and will last up to eight weeks.

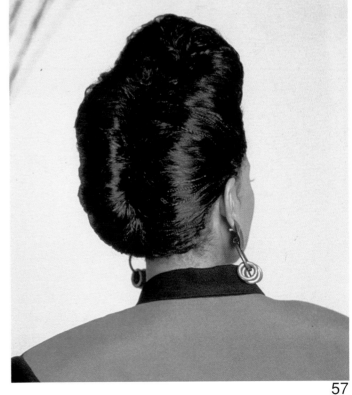

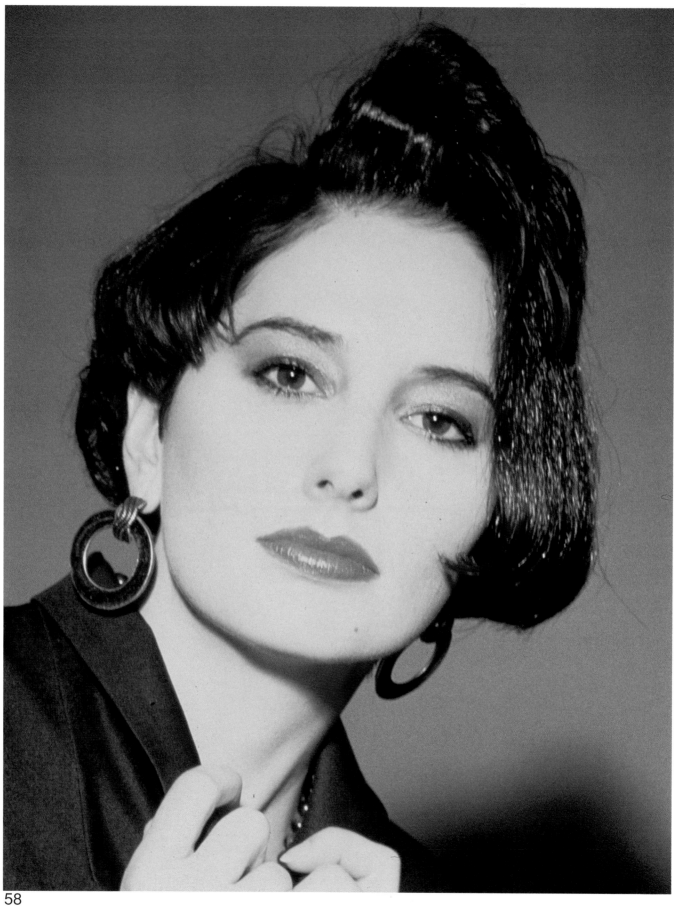

58

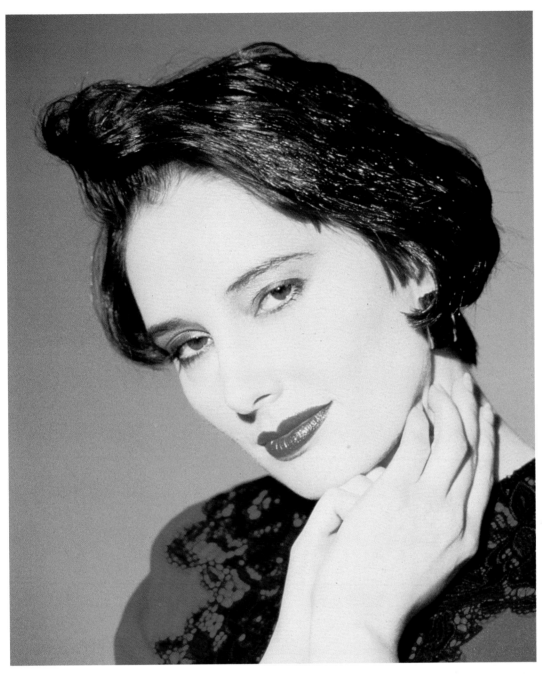

This client's naturally fine hair would not grow long enough for a bob style. Hair extensions were added to give her hair length and volume.

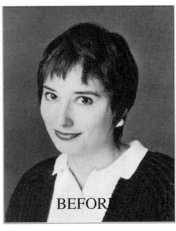

BEFORE

59

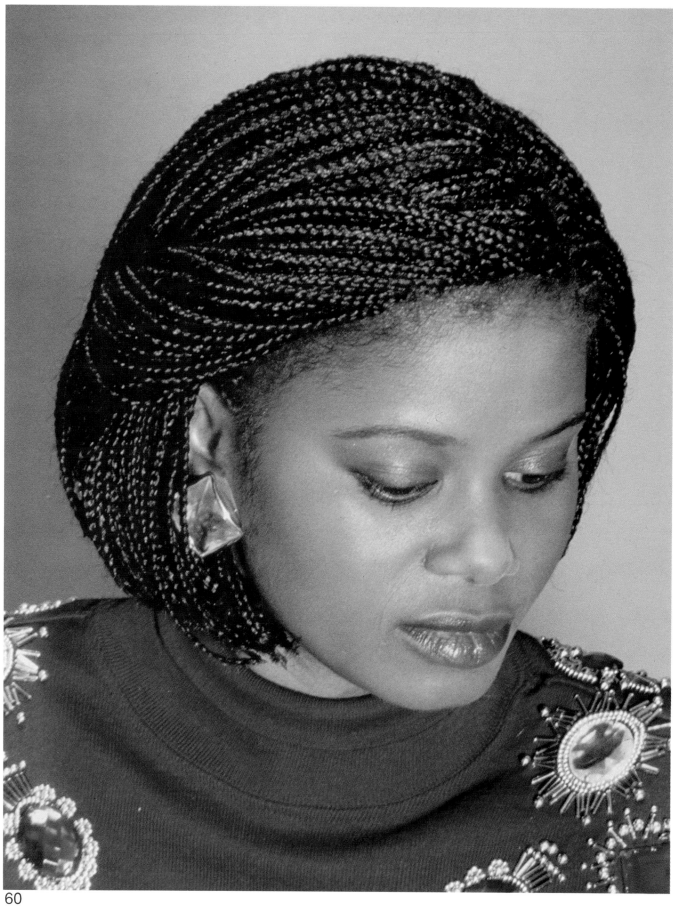

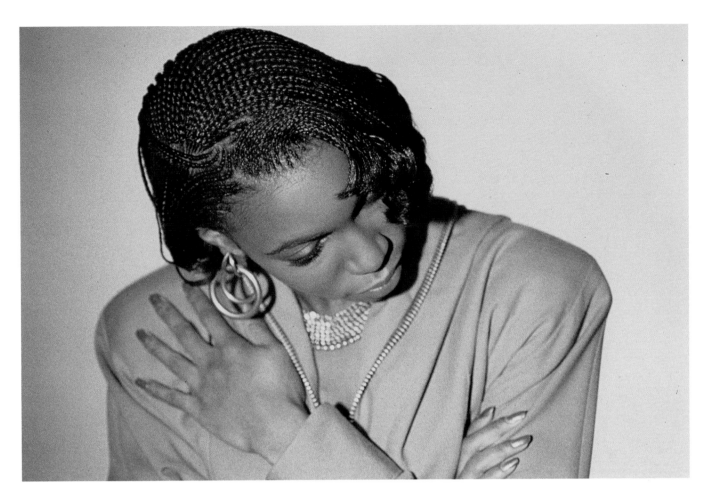

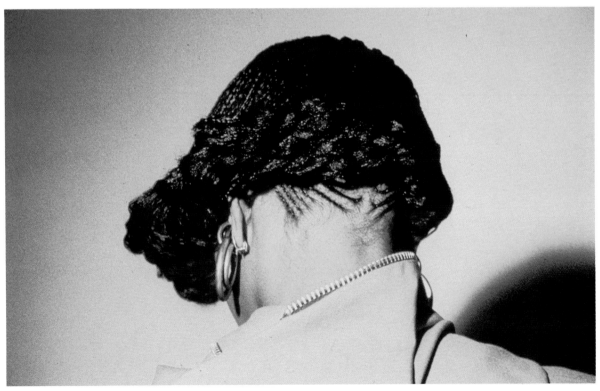

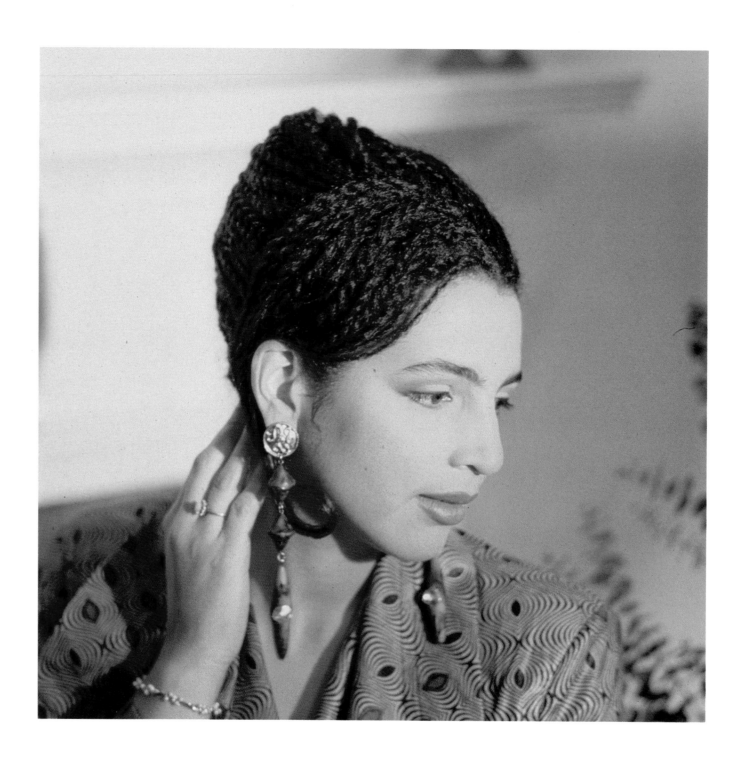

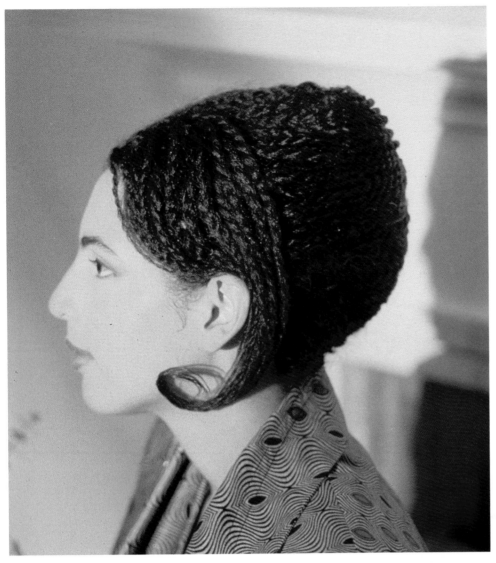

<u>"Twist"</u>
The beauty alternative for natural hair. This style offers easy flexibility and takes only two hours to do.

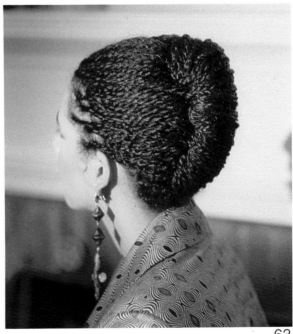

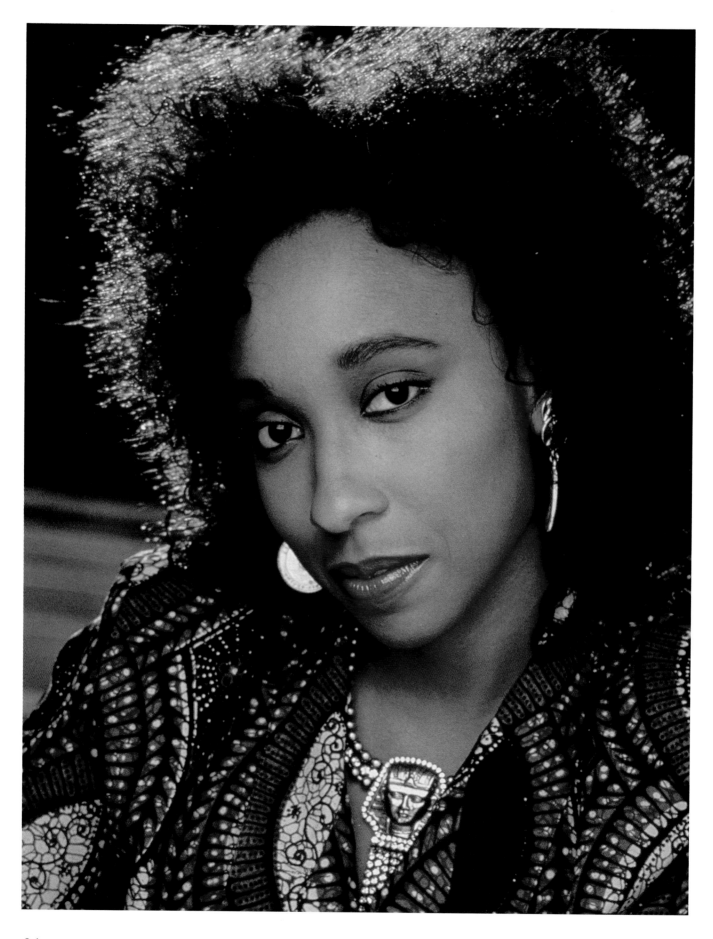

6
Where Style Touches Beauty

Truly beautiful women are most remembered for their physical attributes, character, talents , and style and not necessarily in this order. It should be every woman's desire to be as memorable as possible. And it is every woman's responsibility to discover and develop her innate beauty potential. Taken even further, a truly beautiful woman evolves into her own personal "beauty style." She makes the good visible.

The Audience Society

To open that heavy door of style development we must first dispense with myths and standards engendered by a society of audiences. Because style and beauty standards are not always created by the people that are to uphold them, they are often harsh and unrealistic. In other words, most women cannot live up to the beauty standards and requirements of an audience of people who do not have to fulfill them themselves.

I often see women struggling physically, emotionally, and financially to fashion their physical attributes to meet an impossible criteria. With the fundamental visual guidelines set forth in this book, I hope to make your beauty quest a vacation, rather than an odyssey.

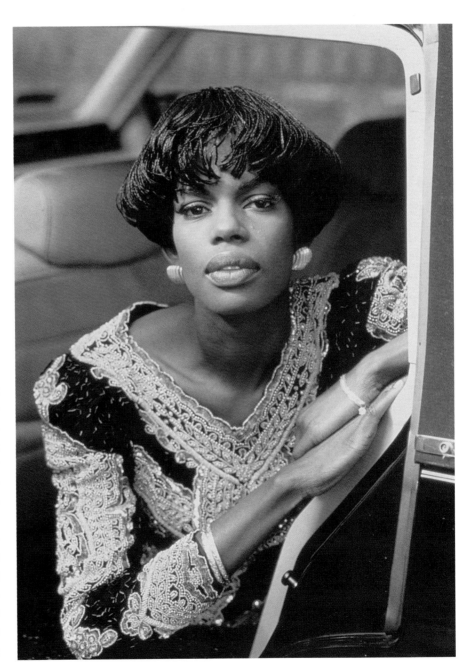

Braid in the USA

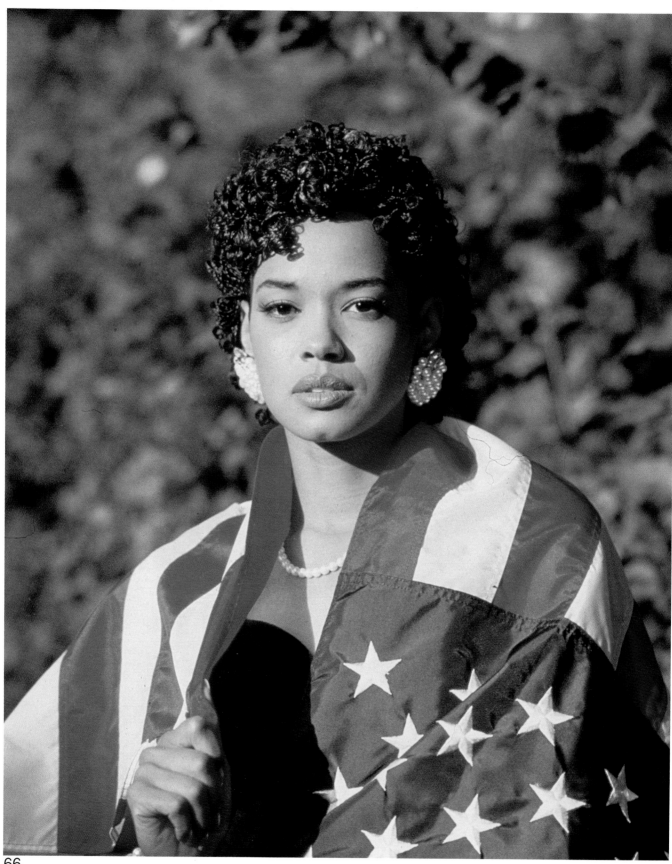

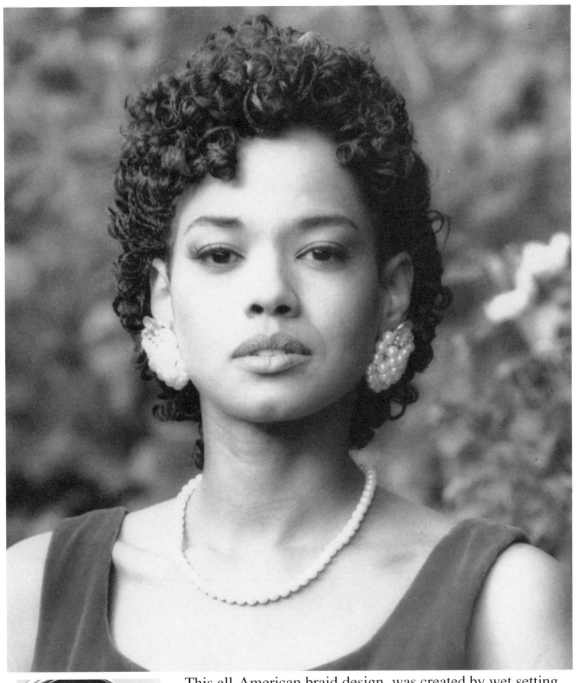

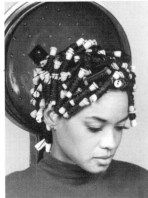

This all-American braid design was created by wet setting human hair individual braids on perm rods. The curls will last until the braids are shampooed.

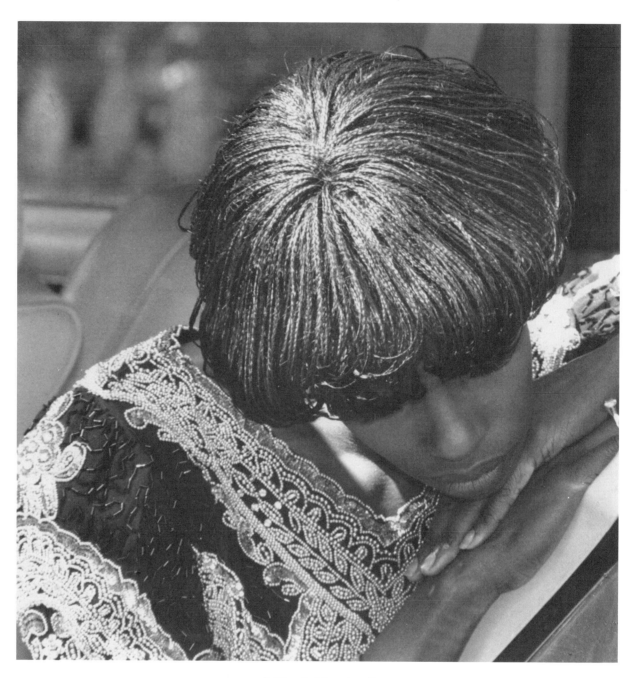

"Sleek Wedge"

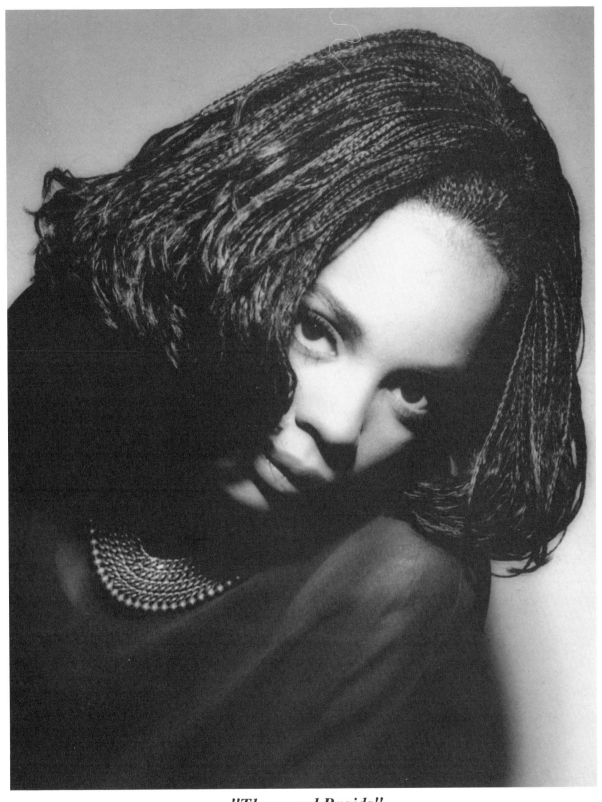

"Thousand Braids"

To create this contemporary style cut, human hair extensions were added to fine individuals braids.

WHAT YOU SEE IS WHAT YOU GET

Before you can develop yourself or solve your beauty problems, you must first identify them. Therefore, the first phase of developing your personal beauty style requires you to take a good look in the mirror. Using a full-length mirror lovingly evaluate all of your beauty components.

Next, mentally and spiritually affirm that you like yourself enough to be willing to develop what you see to its fullest potential. At this point, it is even healthy to talk to yourself in the mirror. Say exactly what you think about what you see and listen to the messages you are sending to yourself. Are you saying, "I hate my hair. I am fat and out of shape. I am ugly and not worth the time and effort?" Or are you saying, "I am beautiful. I have soft, round eyes. I like my hair. I like myself. I will continue to improve all these God-given qualities?"

The second phase is to find your best physical features (i.e., lips, eyes, hair) and accentuate these things. Look at the things that you are not fully satisfied with or that bother you the most and honestly say why you don't like them. Make simple evaluations, for instance, "I don't like my right side profile because my cheekbone structure is weak."

The third phase is to choose styles to diminish your negative features while accentuating the positive. For that weak cheekbone choose a hair style that frames that side of the face, or if you wear a centered hair style, apply makeup to compensate for the weak bone structure. Based on your face shape, facial features, hair condition, body structure, and lifestyle, you can design the style that best suits you.

Face Shapes

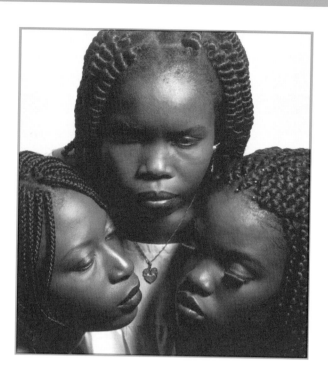

Select your hairstyle based on your face shape

The **Oval face** shape is usually thought of as the perfect face because it is rightly proportioned. Most styles can be worn on this face shape because there are no areas to be minimized or maximized. Keep in mind that an oval face shape can have flaws such as uneven features or special hairline considerations.

The **Oblong face** is generally narrow and long with hollow cheek area. The idea is to make the face look shorter by styling the hair close to the top with a fringe bang. Second, give the illusion that the face is wider by creating a style that is full on the sides, jaw length, and styled behind the ears.

The **Round facial** contour has a round hairline and a round chin line. The objective is to make the face look slender by creating a style that gives the illusion of length. Design your braid style with fullness at the top of the head and arrange the hair over the ears always trying to tone down the roundness. Select a style with straight lines or straight form.

The **Diamond shape** face has a narrow forehead and chin line with extreme width in the cheekbones. The objective is to minimize the width across the cheekbones by styling the hair full across the forehead and jaw line area. Also style the hair coming close to the cheekbones.

The **Square face** is recognized by a straight hairline and square shape jawline. Our aim is to give the illusion of length by styling the hair high and to soften the square corners of the face. If the hair is parted, make a diagonal part and for styles with a center or off center part, the hair should fall through the hairline.

The **Pear shape** face has a narrow forehead, a wide round jawline and chin area. The aim is to make this face shape look proportioned by creating a style that gives the illusion of width at the forehead. Style the top hair full and high while slightly covering some of the forehead with a fringe bang. Style the hair close to the cheeks to soften the wideness and to give balance to the narrow forehead.

The **Heart shape** face has a wide forehead and a slender chin line. Your objective is to minimize the width of the forehead while creating the illusion of width in the chin line area. Create a style that is slanted to one side and cut around the chin line to give softness and width.

These seven basic face shapes will help you create styles that will maximize your weak area while minimizing the overpowering ones. For face shapes that may differ from these seven basic shapes keep in mind the aim is usually to create length or width, add softness and detract the area that makes the face look out of proportion. Your main goal is to create styles that are becoming to you.

FACIAL FEATURES

When selecting a hair style, if your features are proportioned and prefect most styles would be complimenting to the face shape. Unfortunately, many women do not feel that their facial features are perfect, so I have listed simple suggestions for the most common facial feature complaints.

Big/ high forehead---*There are women who often complain about having a big forehead, however, only 5% really have this problem. I tend to believe that the female goes through a phase in her life where she feels comfort in hiding behind a bang. Usually during the adolescent age, a bang becomes a symbol of growing up. It makes the young girl feel older and secure. The adult who fears giving up her bang has many times had childhood conditioning that her forehead was big and she should never show it.*

For the 5% women that really have this problem a full or side bang works well to minimize the wide protruding "big forehead." Fringing the bang gives softness and is recommended for the female with small facial features. A side bang is good if you are trying to come out of a bang style or need to slenderize the forehead area.

Low forehead is where the hairline grows close to the outer edge of the eyebrow. Style the hair away from the face. To wear a bang style the hair off center with a little lift to give the forehead the illusion of length.

Protruding ears can be camouflage by styling the hair close to the face to cover the ears completely or by styling the hair directly behind the ears with some fullness to cover the top of them.

Uneven Features can be balanced by designing a style that is not centered. A balanced style requires both sides to be identical. Style the hair off center aiming to achieve evenness.

Wide Flat Nose can be minimized by creating a style where the hair is away from the face, since this nose shape makes the face appear broader. Hair styles with natural texture are always more becoming than straightened hair.

Short Fat Neck or double chin will appear slender by styling the crown with height and creating the nape area to look tapered.

Long Neck a symbol of beauty in certain parts of Africa. If you feel self conscious about your long neck avoid styling the hair up from the back of the head.

There are many imperfections and beauty flaws that can be easily disguised by designing a hair style to minimize the problem. However, obesity, bad skin, crooked and rotten teeth, halitosis or a nasty attitude are some of the things that a hair style cannot conceal.

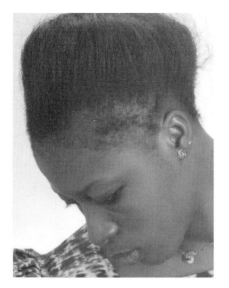
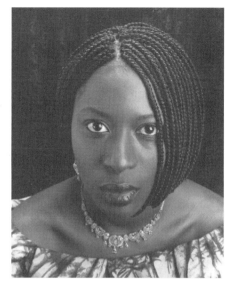

Weak thin/bald hairline---*style the hair to cover the hairline so that you do not continue to put stress on that area. Avoid relaxing the hairline or pulling it tight with braids.*

DESIGNING A STYLE FOR YOUR HAIR......

Hair texture, condition, and length play a major part in style design. Some women are limited to wearing certain hair styles because their natural hair condition may not support others. However, many women are confined to a particular hair style because they have abused their hair where the hairline is permanently bald, the crown is thin, the ends are straggly and limp from chemical over processing, or the hair lengths are uneven due to hair breakage. When creating a braid style, the face shape and hair condition should be considered.

Thin Crown area---Avoid hair styles that part down the middle. Design the style to braid through the thin area so that it gives good coverage or creates a style that is full over this area. Up styles also work well to cover this condition and they do not add stress to that area.

Thin straggly limp ends ---Most braid styles with extensions will hide this problem, allowing the hair to grow out so that the ends can be gradually cut off. If you are styling your hair without extensions, depending on the length, style the hair in a secure pin-up style that requires no combing or exposing the ends.

Naturally kinky hair is perfect for braiding, twisting, locking and styling. This hair type is flexible, versatile and easy to manage with the proper styling tools and knowledge.

Straight hair textures both naturally and relaxed are the most difficult hair types to braid because the hair is slippery, not as pliable as curly/kinky hair, and hard to grip. When braiding straight hair it should not be newly cut. Braiding straight hair wet makes it flexible and easier to grasp.

Damaged uneven hair requires corrective styling. If you are wearing the hair with no extensions, cut the hair down to the shortest length creating a style that compliments the face shape.

Hair extensions are a solution for uneven hair because the extension will add length and fullness to where it is needed.

Dandruff and itchy scalp--- the best style for this scalp condition is individual braids or a weekly twist style. These styles allow you to easily cleanse and massage the scalp area as often as needed.

LIFE STYLE DICTATES HAIR STYLE.....

What you do in your day-to-day life, where you work, and how you perceive yourself dictate your hair style. The essentials for a good hair design are its functionality, appropriateness and cost to upkeep it. As the saying goes, "Cost is no object," but in all practicality choose a natural or braid style that you can afford to maintain and keep looking fresh. That style should be functional for work and leisure.

Low budget lifestyle... the college student, housewife, or woman who is on a restricted budget should not use this as a reason to neglect her hair care and hair style. Cornrow styles that take up to four hours and last for two months are a good investment. Natural hair styles such as a "fro," locks, and twists (see chapter 3) are attractive, and low budget.

Disabled lifestyle ---Children, handicapped, pregnant women, and convelscents all need hair care and hair styles that do not require daily combing. Braided hair styles are best suited for the disabled lifestyle, because they are healthy for the hair, easy to care for, and attractive without the fuss. My clients who have severe arthritis, small children, blindness or conditions which make it difficult to groom the hair have found this style choice to be perfect for their needs.

Active lifestyle---if your schedule is such that you do not have the time to go to the salon frequently, you exercise, swim, and do activities that require wetting the hair often, individual braids are recommended This style of braids is durable and versatile enough to withstand the wear and tear of the active woman.

Professional Lifestyle ---this woman is not exempt from wearing braid styles. She should select a braid style based on her dress. For a very uniform/conservative image choose cornrow styles that are pin-ups such as a chignon, french roll, or simple cornrow. If you would like a contemporary braid style cut, with the flexibility to curl it choose between individual braids, lacing, and interlock. Most importantly the corporate woman's braid style must be immaculate and well groomed at all times. Corporate means neat, it does not mean shedding what is culturally yours (kinky hair or African inspired braid styles) to adopt an image (i.e straightened hair) that will cause you hair problems.

Independent lifestyle---the artist, or woman that is in a creative and individualistic business environment. She has a lot of variety and flexibility in the braid or natural hair styles she wears. I encourage her to try many looks and find one that suits her personality.

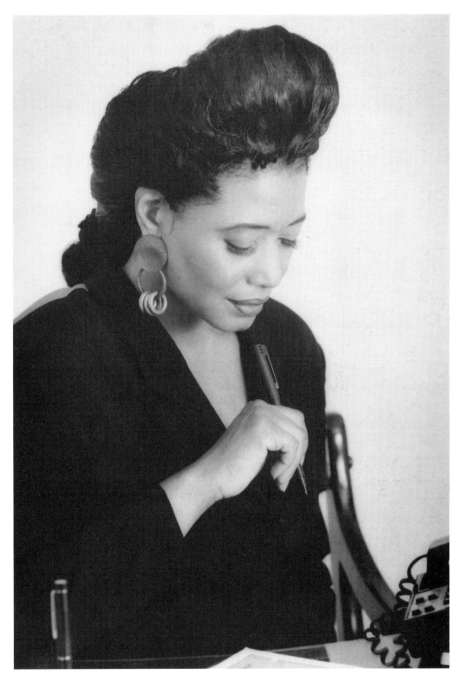

Lace braids are a popular choice for the professional lifestyle.

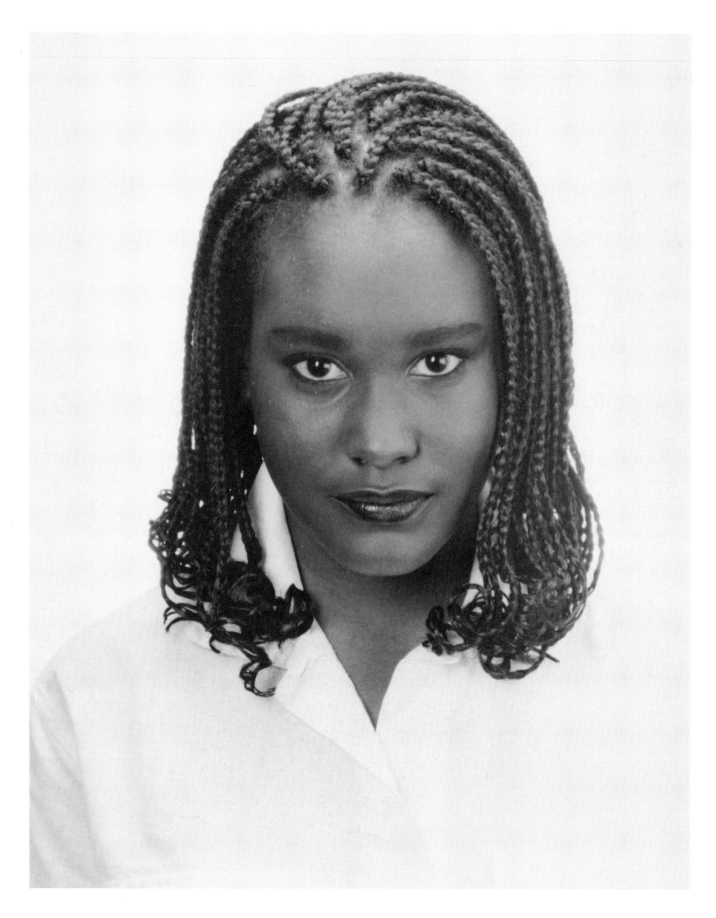

74

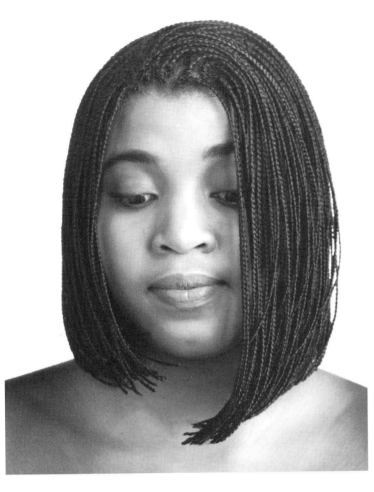

Individual Braids

For unlimited style options and a lasting effect, individual braids with synthetic extensions are a favorable choice.

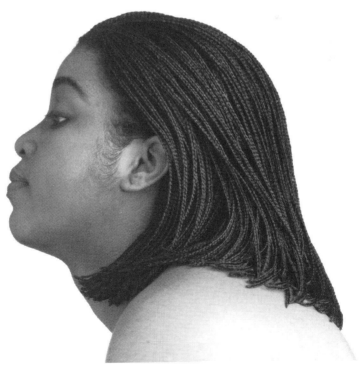

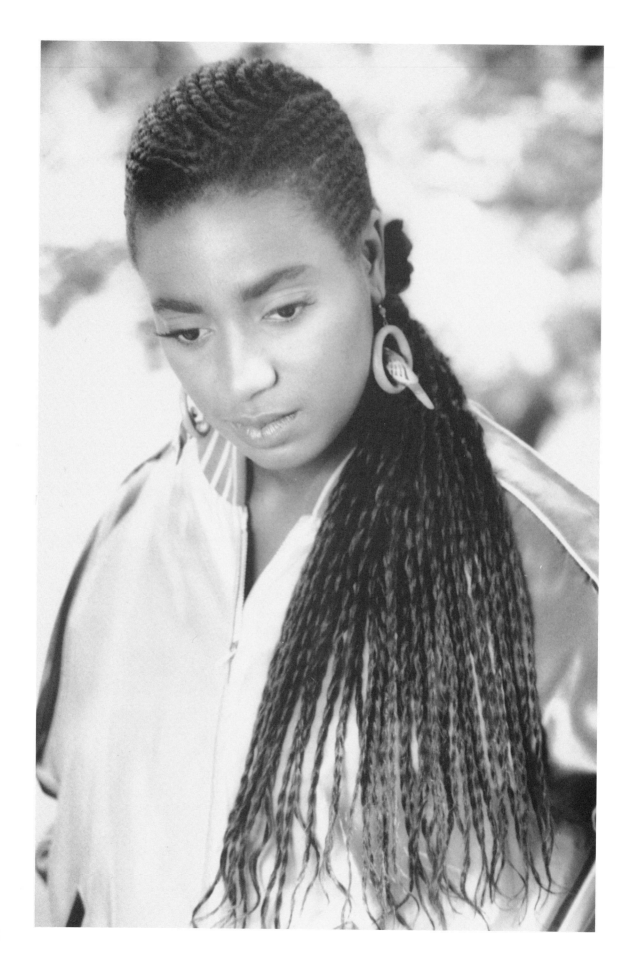

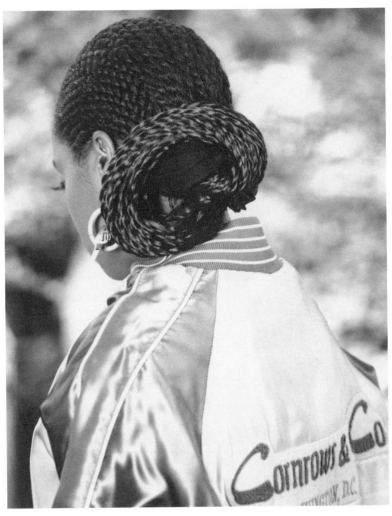

"Long Flat Twist"

Quick and casual ponytail hanging or pinned up for a classic look. The flat twist style takes only one hour to do and will last up to one week.

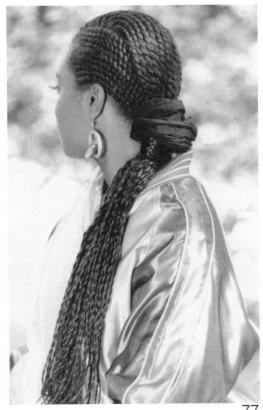

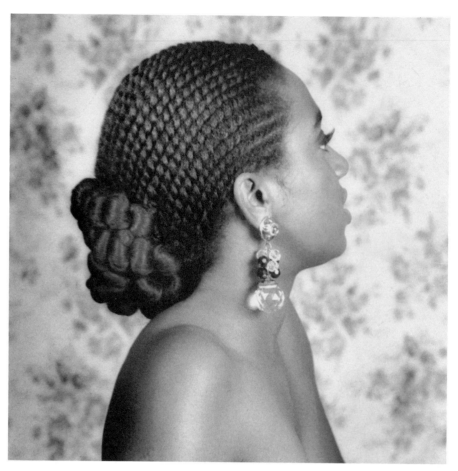

"Soft Sculpted Chignon"
For texture definition lin fiber was added to the ends
of this clients flat twist .

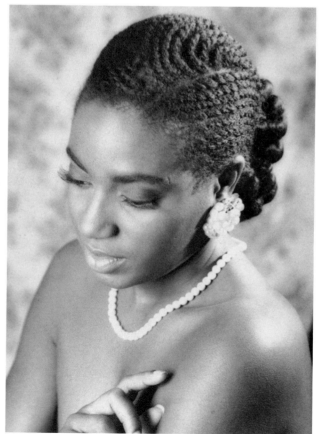

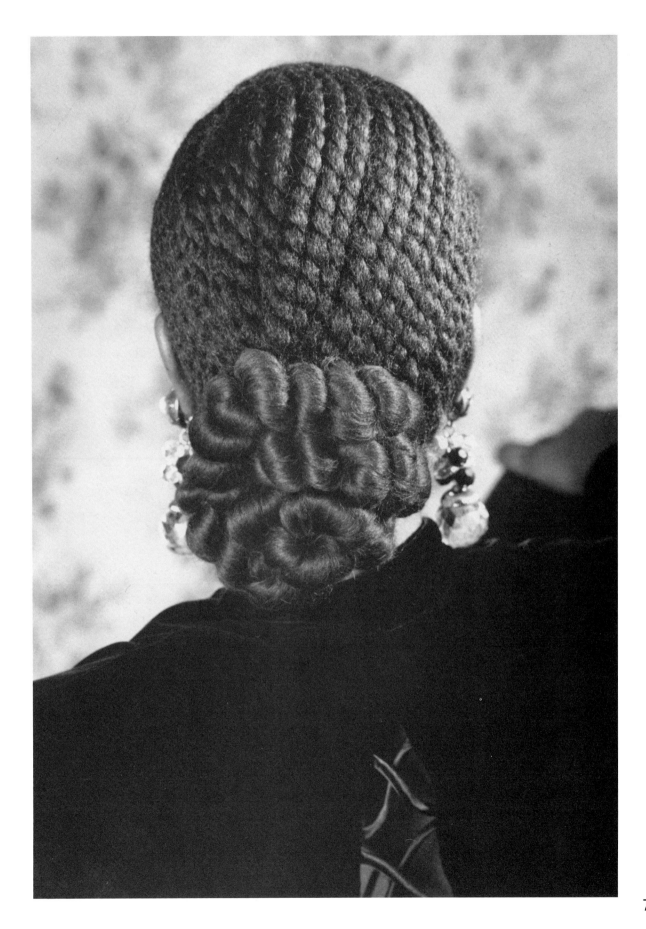

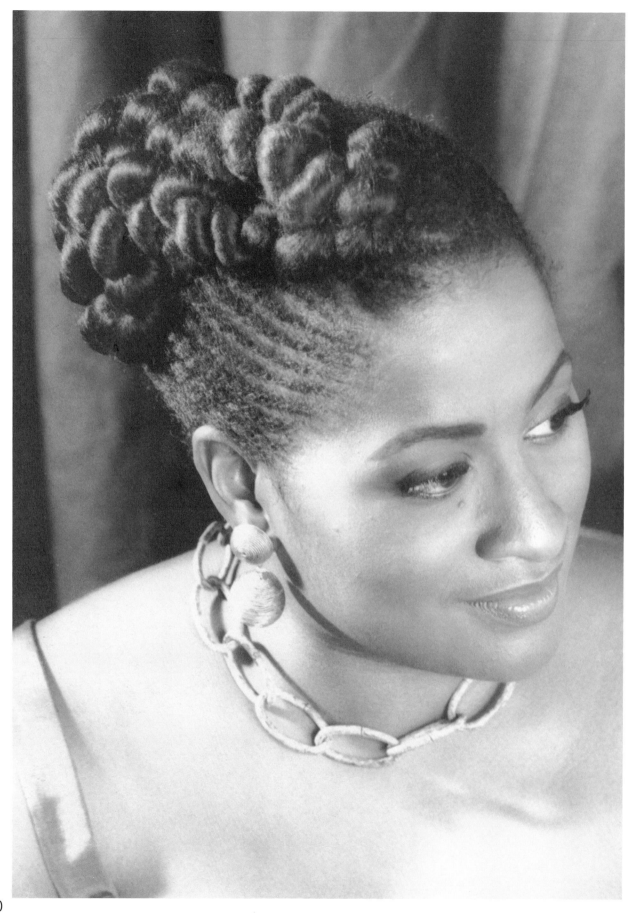

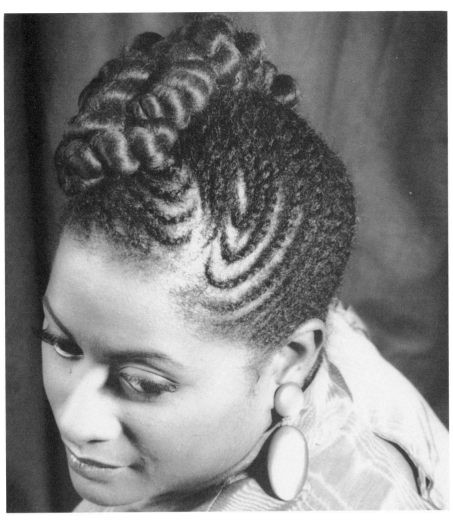

"Popcorn"

*An artstyle of mixed media.
Lin fiber ncorporated into soft
circular flat twist design.*

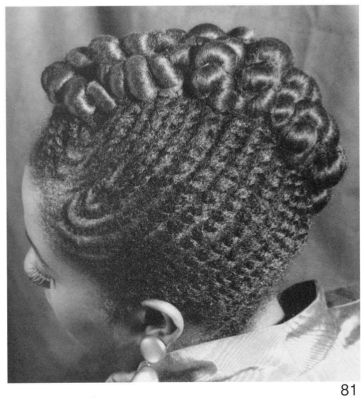

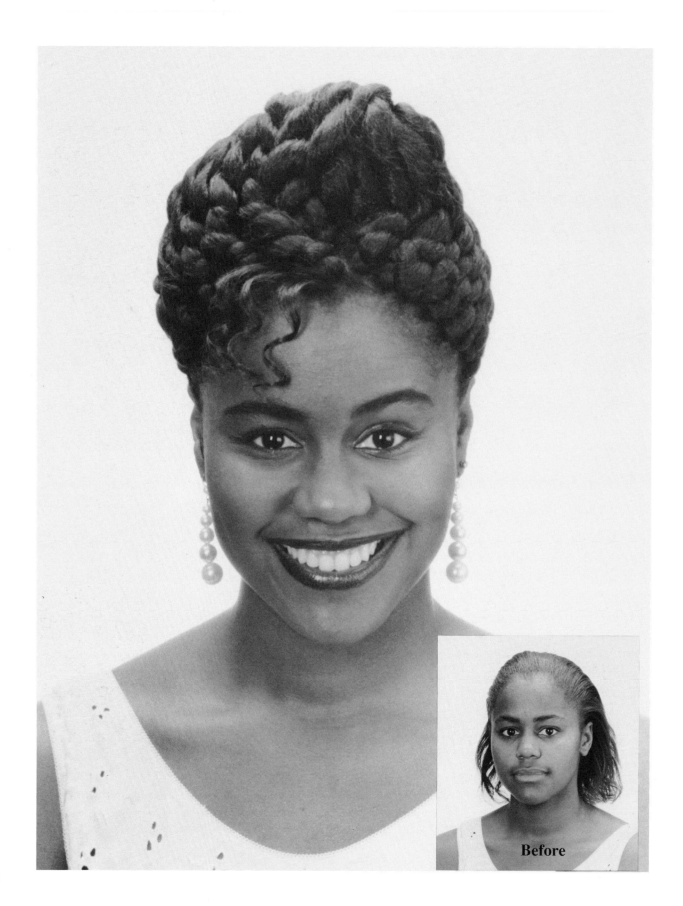

Before

82

Braid Beauty Solutions

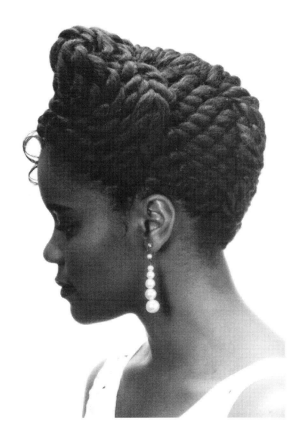
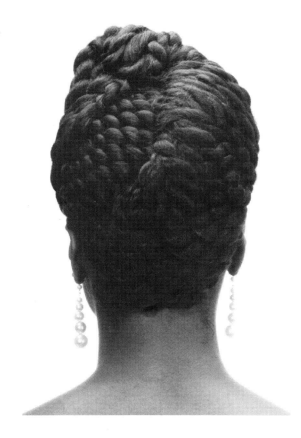

"Soft Twist"

Lin extension was added to this client's flat twist to create a soft full effect. This style takes two hours to do and will last up to two weeks.

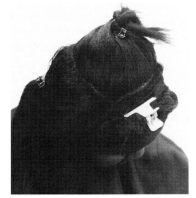
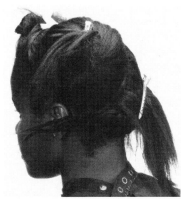
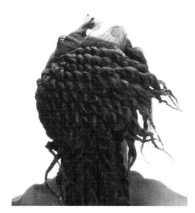

1. Divide the hair into 3 sections. Part from the left neckline on a diagonal up to the front horizontal part.

2. Flat twist with lin extension across the neck hairline. Twist the two back sections to meet at the middle diagonal part.

3. Flat twist the front section from the hairline to meet at the crown part. To finish, gather the ends of the twist creating a diagonal French roll in the back and a beehive in the front.

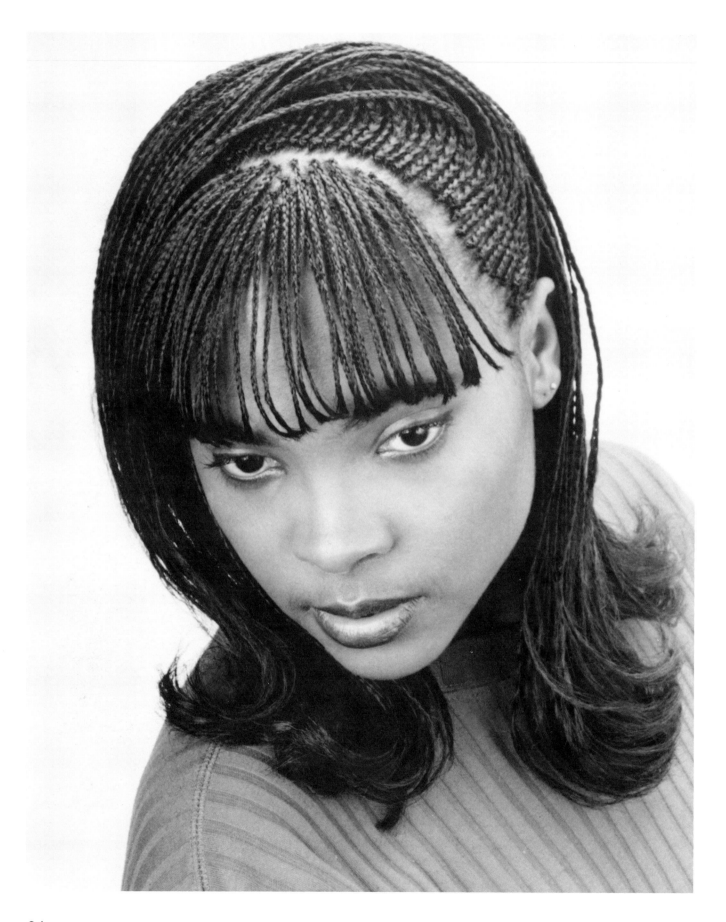

84

"Braid Flip"

The best of two worlds, a hairstyle with straight lines without having to straighten your hair. To protect this client's damaged hair we added human hair extension to create a look of sleekness. This style was designed with individuals in the back and cornrows across the front crown.

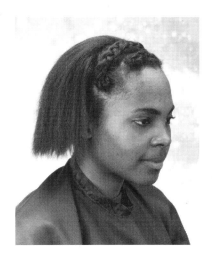

1. Divide the hair into 3 sections. **a)** small 2" bang area **b)** a 3" section across the top front area. **c)** the back area which makes up 3/4 of the head.

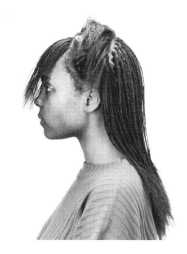

3. Individually braid the bang area using short thin pieces of human hair extension.

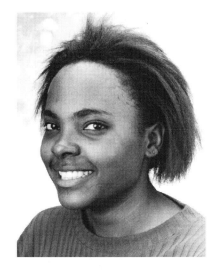

Before

Preparation: 1/2 pound of human hair extension, clips, scissors, comb, large size electric curling irons.

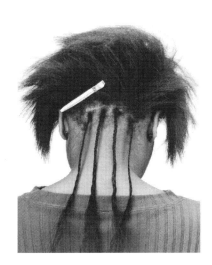

2. Using thin pieces of human hair extension begin individually braiding at the nape area up to the crown of the head.

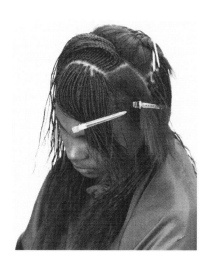

4. Cornrow the top middle section starting from the left side working across to the right side. *To finish; curl the ends of the braids upward and the bang section under.*

85

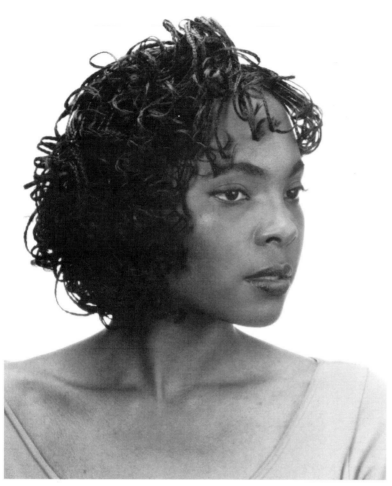

For a different style tightly curl the "Braid Flip". (page 84)

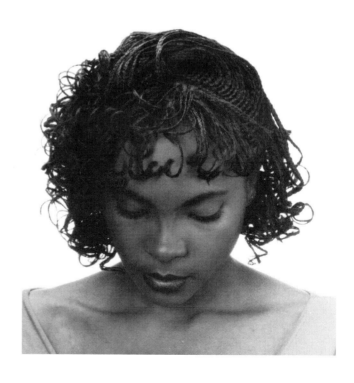

"Gala Fringe"

Gayle, who enjoys her natural, wanted a short braid style. To create a feeling of height while complimenting her beautiful eyes, the braids were shaped to frame the face. We then styled the back braids to blend into her tapered neckline.

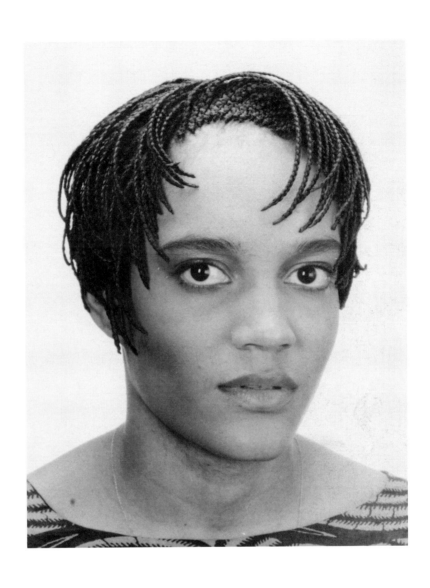

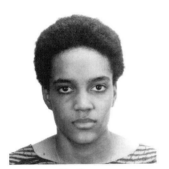

Before

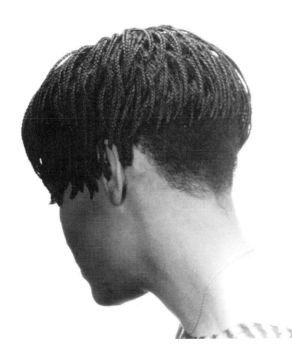

Four easy steps to complete this six hour braid style. The tight stitch braid makes the permanant curved shape and will remain neat up to two months. Perfect for swimming and frequent shampooing.

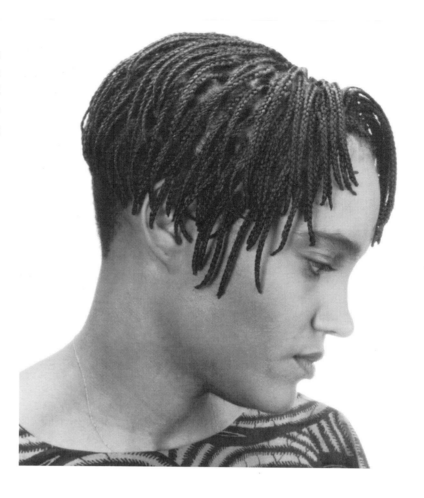

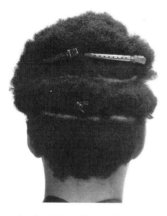

1. Part the hair into 3 sections. (The bottom section will be cut close to the neckline).

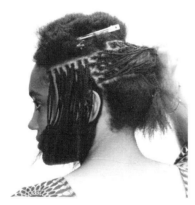

2. Using small pieces of extension, tight stitch individually braid the middle and top sections .

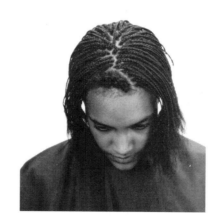

3. Cornrow the small section in the front in diagonal direction off the hairline to create lift.

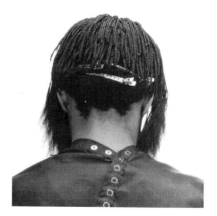

4. To seal the ends of the braids, burn the synthetic extension 1/4" below the natural hair in different lengths to give a layered affect. Cut the back nape area.

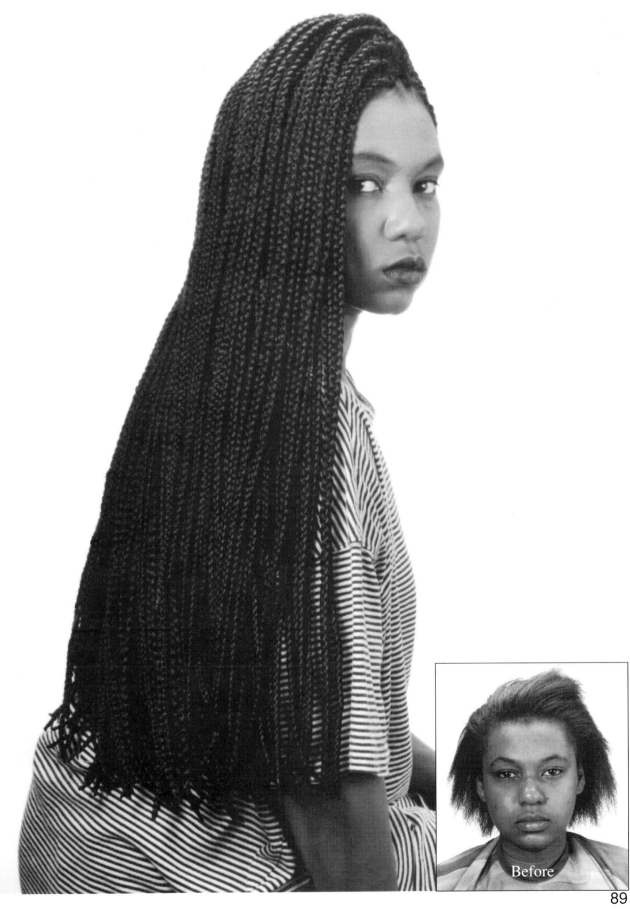

Before

89

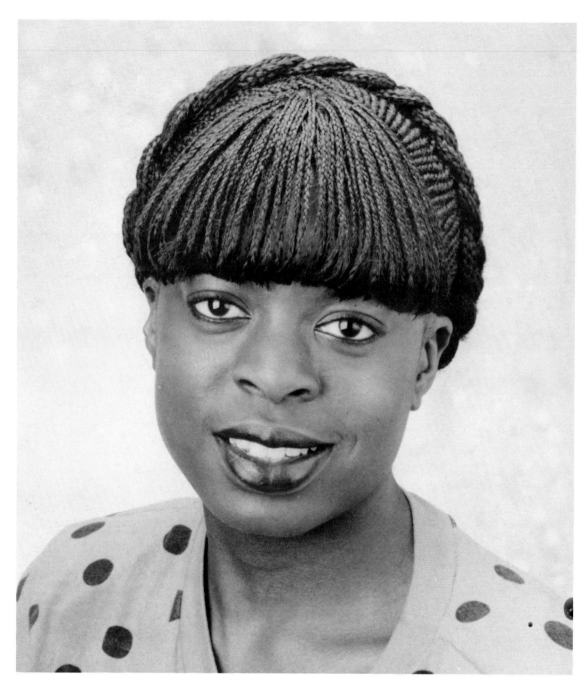

"CORNROW CROWN"

An African inspired corporate look offers a refreshing change for this client's permed hair. This style takes up to four hours and will last eight weeks.

Preparation: 2 packs of synthetic fiber, clips, mediun curling irons, scissors.

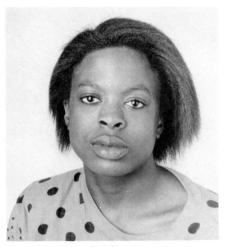

Before

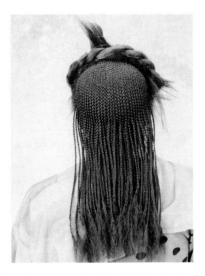

2. Cornrow the back layer down through the neck line.

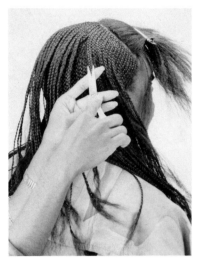

4. Cornrow the front section back off the face. Clip the frizzy hair from the braids to give a neat finished look.

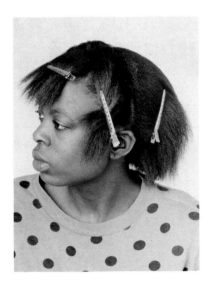

1. Section the hair from ear to ear across the crown of the head. Part a half circle along the front hairline for the bang.

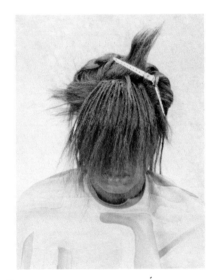

3. Individually braid the bang using fine pieces of extension.

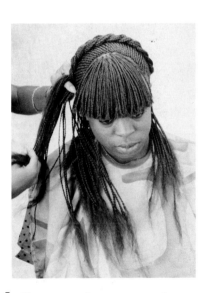

5. To create the cornrowed crown, braid the ends of the cornrows together around the back of the head.

To finish; secure the braid ends and pin the large cornrow into a flat circle. Curl the bang under.

91

THICK ROWS

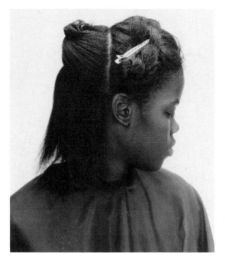

1. Divide the hair into three sections.

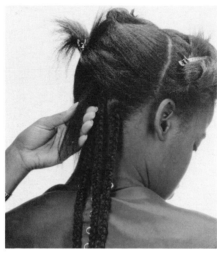

2. At the neck line part a 1" round section for thick braids.

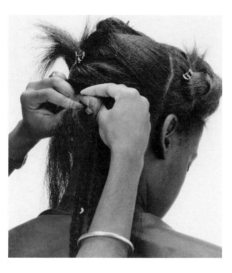

3. Underhand braid large pieces of extension into the natural hair.

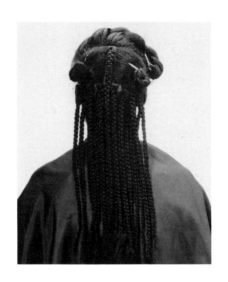

4. Cornrow the second section, starting in the middle, working out to the sides.

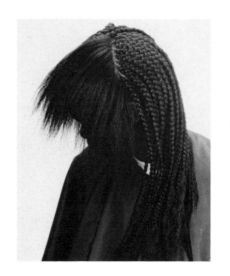

5. Cornrow the front side section down over the ears.

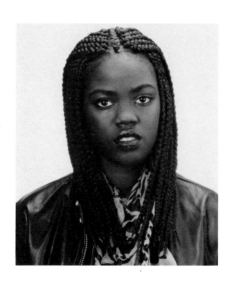

6. Cornrow the top section slanting off the face. To seal the ends, burn with a butane lighter.

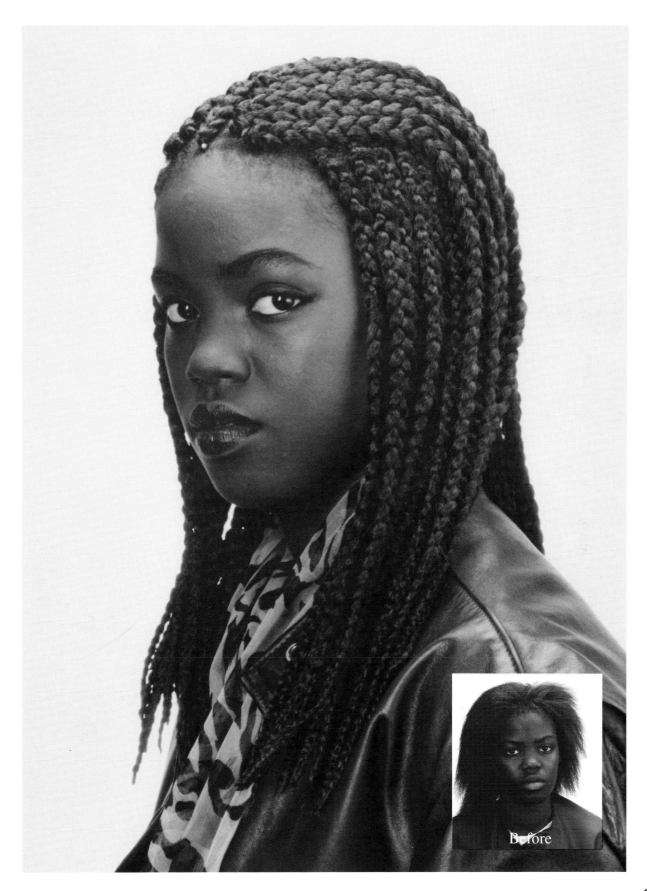

Before

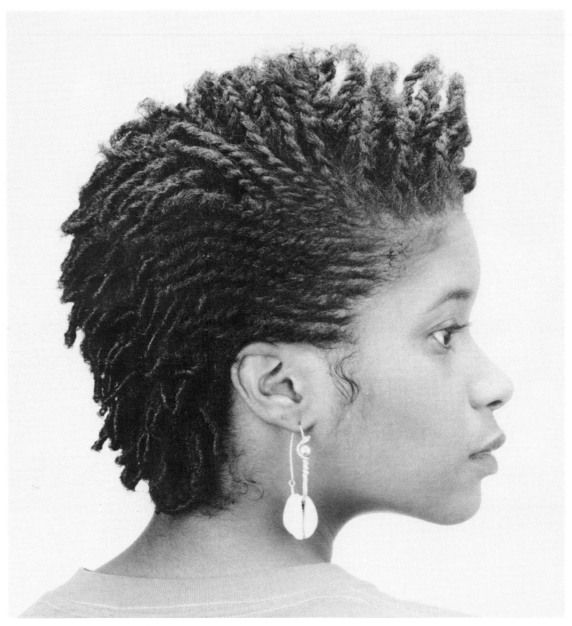

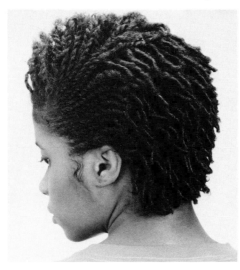

94

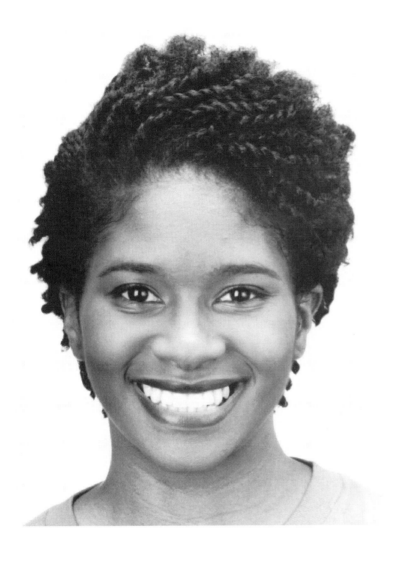

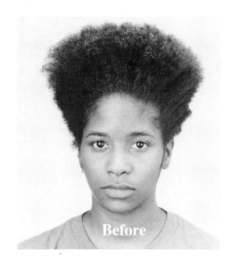

Before

"Twist Rolls"
The frustration of growing your hair out of a short cut is the "in between" length. To give this client a soft textured style, I twist rolled her thick natural hair. This style can take up to three hours and will last up to two weeks or until the hair is shampooed.

Preparation:
This style works best on damp hair. Let the hair partially air dry after shampooing.
Tools: Spray bottle, clips, all purpose comb, hair gel or hair spray.

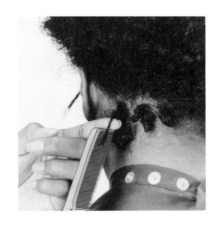

1. Make 1/2" sections; insert the comb to the end of the hair then wind the hair to the end.

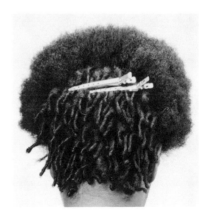

2. Clamp that section flat and spray the hair with a holding spray. Flat twist the sides off the face.

95

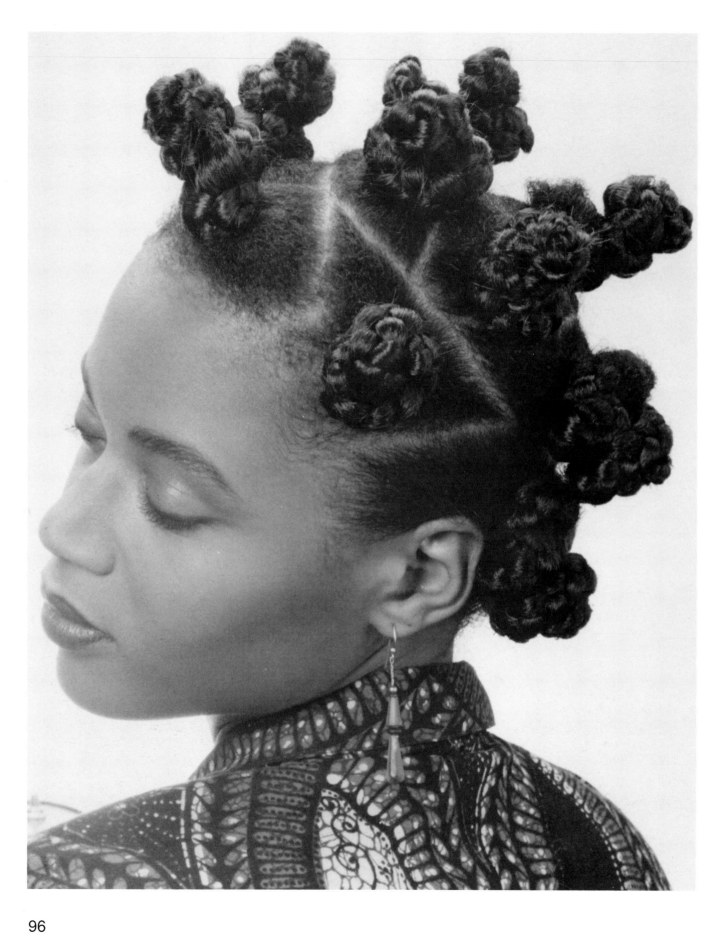

"Nubian Knots"

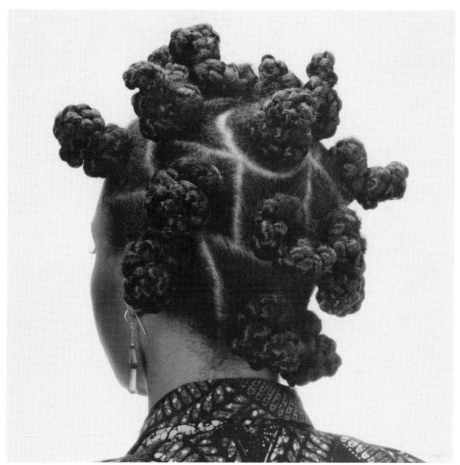

"Controlled Naturalism"
This two dimensional sculptured artstyle integrates the past with the present.

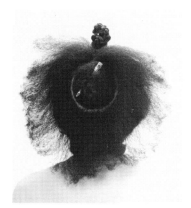

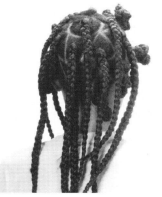

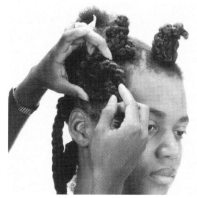

1. Section the hair into 3 horizontal circles around the head.

2. Part triangle sections into each circle, then individually thick braid each section.

3. To create the knot, gently tie each braid 3 times and tuck the ends into the middle.

"URBAN LOCKS"

This client's chiselled features and perfect round head shape is the perfect palette to create a modern rendition of the Nigerian thread wrap. I wrapped a four strand braid with synthetic fiber to transform her short natural into an *"Exotic Artstyle"*. This style can take up to two hours to complete.

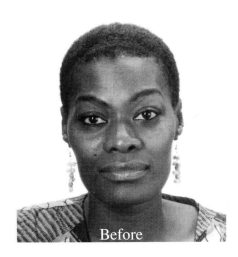

Before

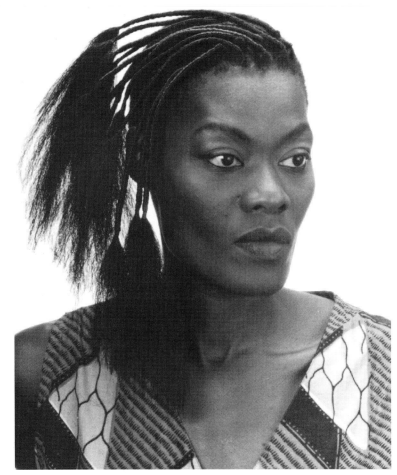

"Bush locks"

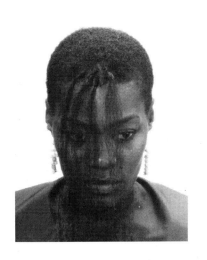

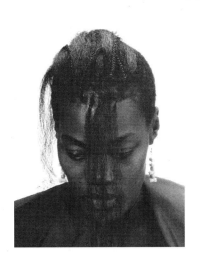

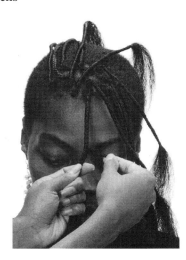

1. Section a round bang area. Begin adding very small amounts of synthetic extension leaving the end loose 1/2" beyond the natural hair.

2. Add a piece of synthetic extension to the middle of two of the extended braids to create a four strand braid.

3. Leave a small piece of hair extension free to wrap around the braid. Seal the end of the wrapped braid with heat.

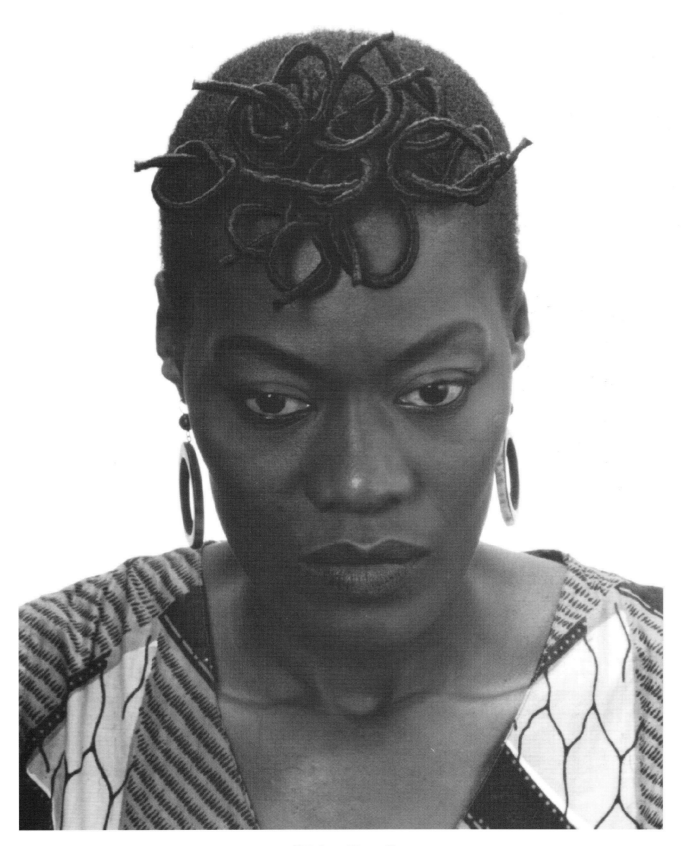

"Urban Knots"

"Daughter Of The Dust"

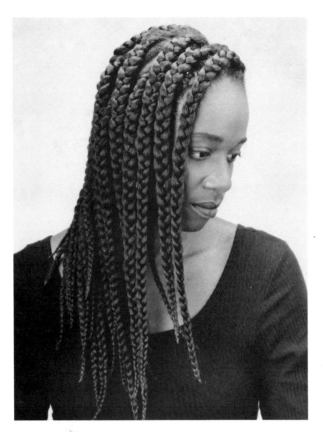

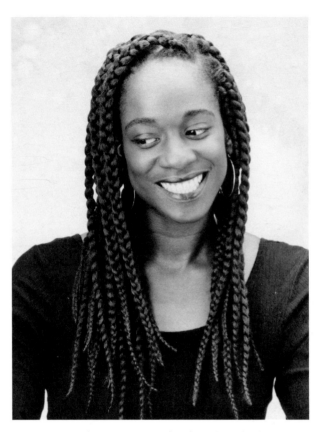

Full textured thick braids offer a quick style that requires little time and low maintenance to enjoy it. A healthy beauty alternative for this late spring model.

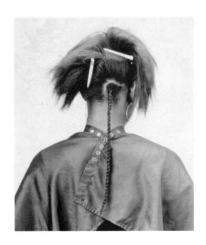

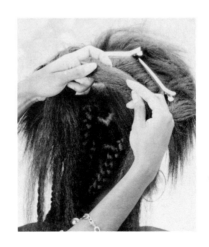

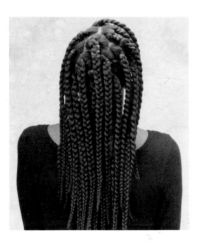

1. Begin at the nape area making a braid that will serve as the guide for the length and size of all the braids.

2. Part a 2" round section and integrate the hair extension by using the over-hand braid technique. This method gives the braid a natural beginning base.

3. Braid the ends thin and burn the tips to seal it closed.

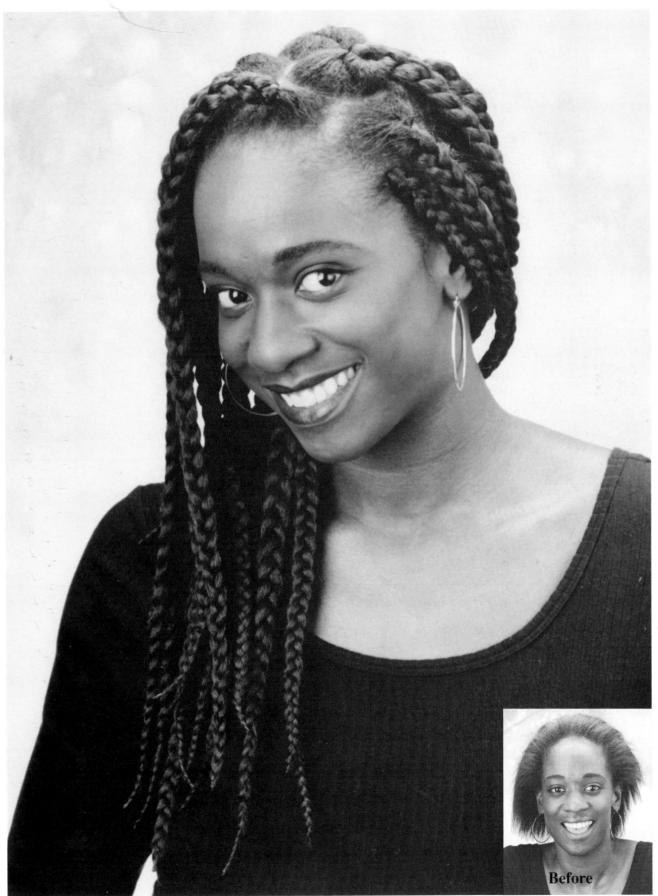

Before

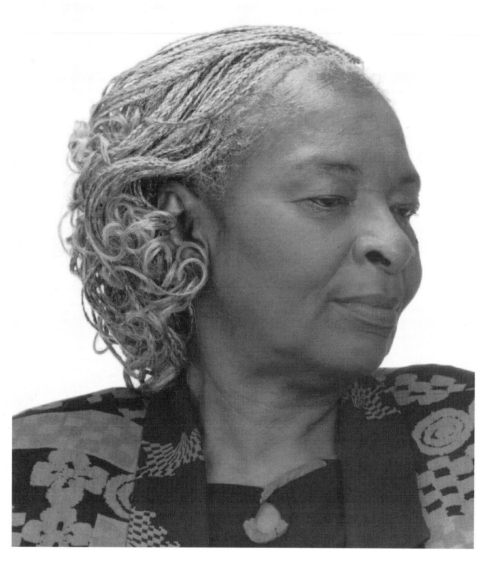

"Silver Lining"

This late Autumn client has a beauty style of her own.
I wet set the braids to give her a long lasting curl and unlimited
style flexibility. Individual braids are the perfect compliment to
her natural silver hair.

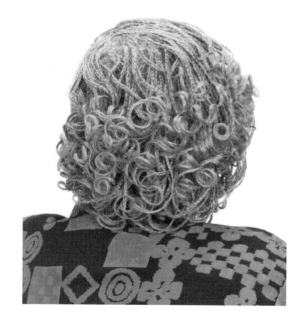

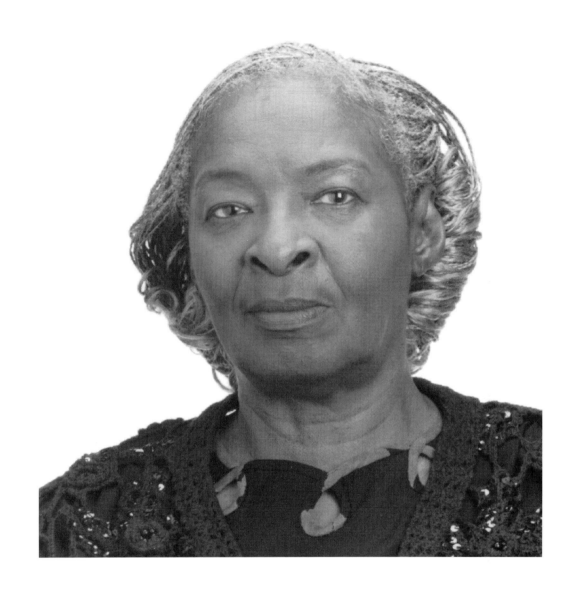

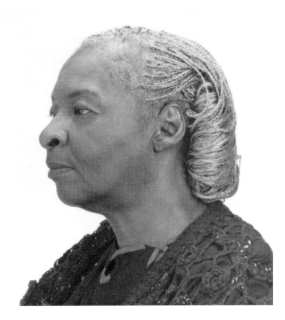

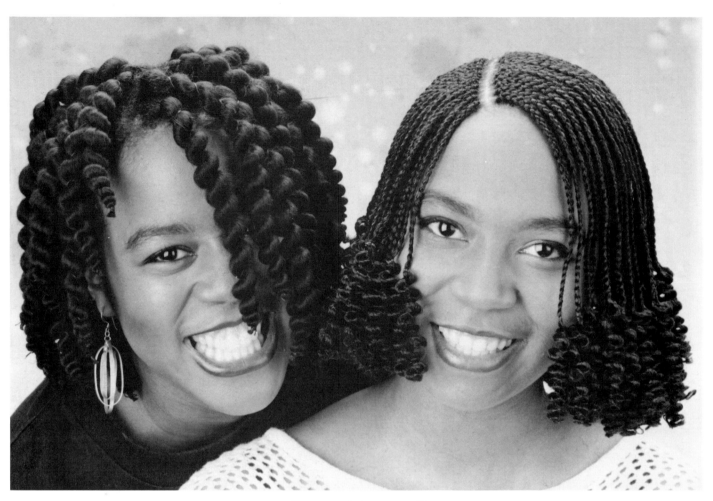

"Double Joy"

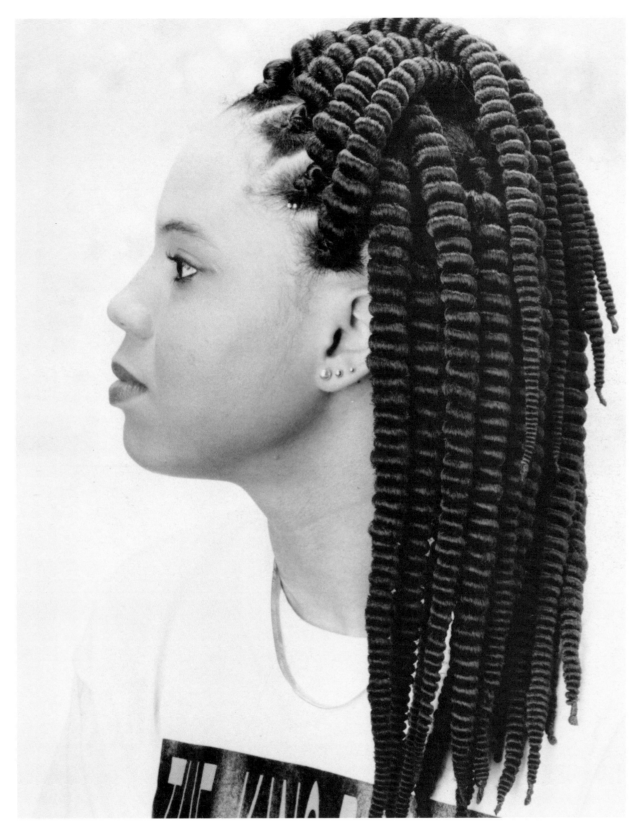

"Corkscrew"

Using the dufil method, (page 107) a synthetic extension was added to give this style longevity. The corkscrew style will last up to eight weeks.

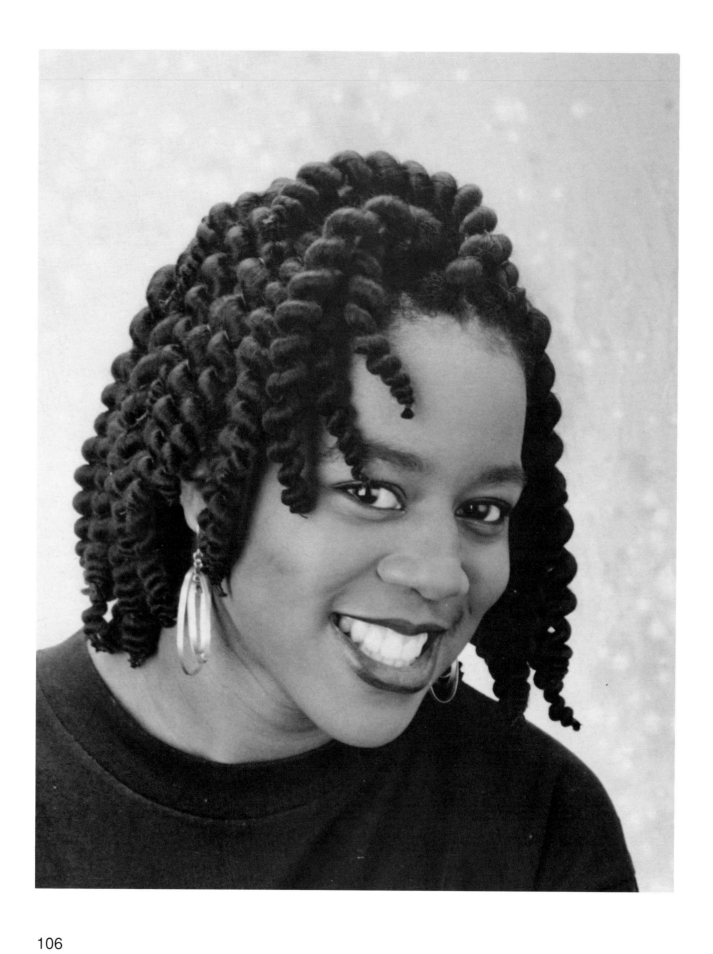

"DUFIL BOB"

Preparation: This style works best on naturally coarse hair.

Tools: Lin hair extension, heavy cotton thread, scissors, clips and combs.

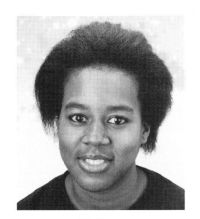

Before

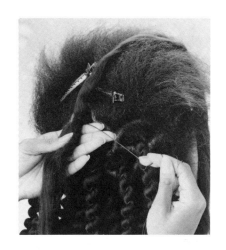

2. Center the lin close to the scalp and wrap securely with heavy cotton thread.

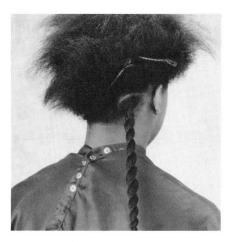

4. In a spiral motion wrap the thread loosely around the lin; descending smaller towards the end.

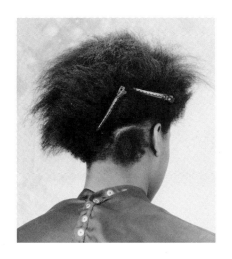

1. Start at the neckline area by sectioning a 2" rounded section.

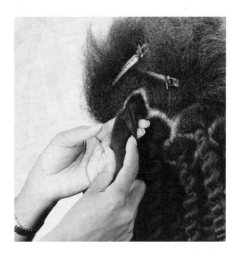

3. Sandwich the natural hair between the lin extension.

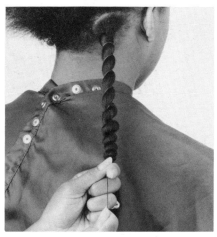

5. Hold the thread in one hand and the lin in the other. Push the lin upward toward the scalp while holding the thread stationary. Seal the ends with a triple tie knot.

"CURLY BOB"

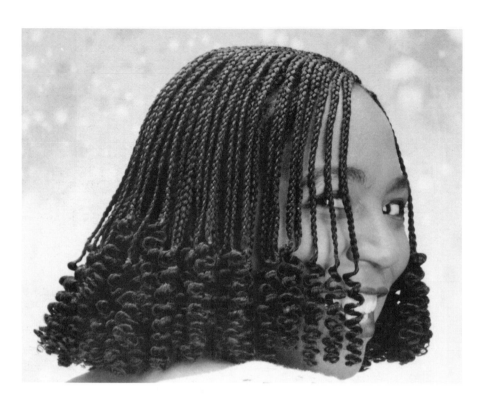

A contemporary bob with an ancient twirl. Layers of corn-rows attain a look of balance. To create the full curly ends, whole African curls were separated. This style will remain neatly braided and curly up to eight weeks. Looks great on a round or square face shape and is a healthy style for a thinning weak hairline.

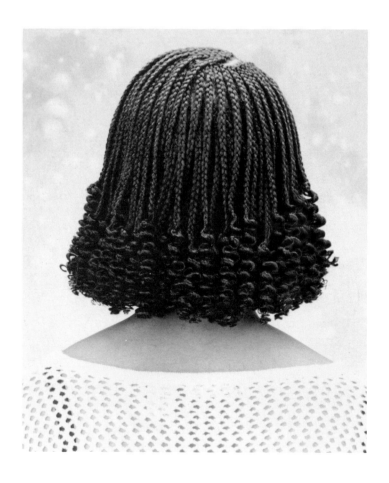

108

PREPARATION:

Shampoo, condition and blow dry the hair.

Tools: Comb, clips, 3-4 packs of synthetic fiber, small tea pot (to boil water), heavy black cotton thread, 6 fluffy towels (to protect the shoulders from hot dripping water) .

*(**Note:** The African curl should only be done by a skilled braider .)*

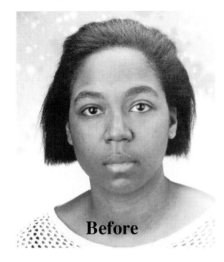

Before

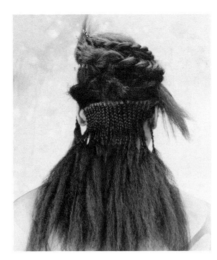

2. Establish a guide for the length of the braids. Cornrow each layer ending the braid 1/4" beyond the length of the natural hair. Leave the extension ends loose to create the African curl.

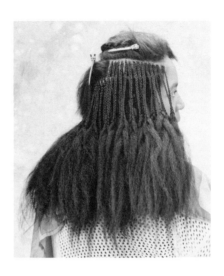

4. Cornrow the top layer from the front side part angling the braids to fall in the face. To finish the ends, create an African curl starting with the bottom layer. Gather 3-4 braids: wrap and secure a double thread around the top of the loose hair, then do the same method as the Dufil. (see page 107)

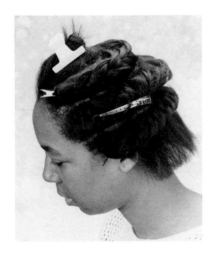

1. Part the hair into 5 horizontal layers then twist loosely each layer to keep the hair separated as you braid.

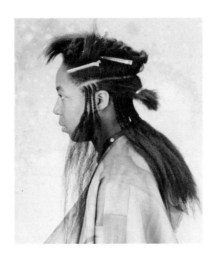

3. Continue braiding the second layer starting at the front left side working around to the front right side.

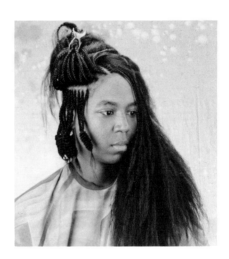

5. Dip the African curl in hot water for 2 seconds. Let the excess water drip on several towels. Blow dry the curl with warm air. Clip the thread wrapped ends and carefully remove the thread from the curl. To create the curly ends, separate the 4-5 braids within the African curl.

109

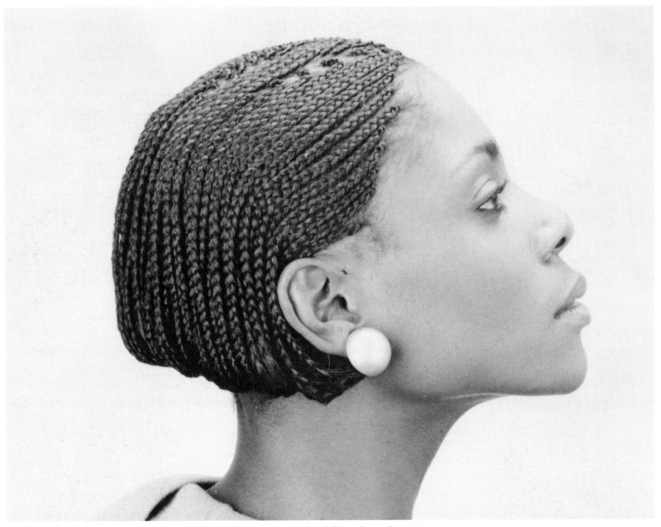

The "Ancient records of Khemet" confirm the idea that there is nothing new under the sun. This clients strong Nubian features are a distinct reminder of the history of our beauty.

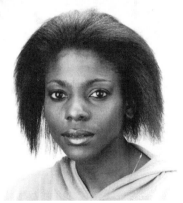

Before

110

"Ancient Wedge"

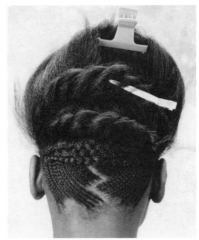

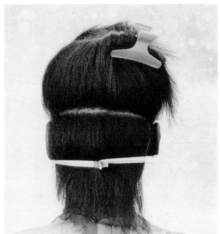

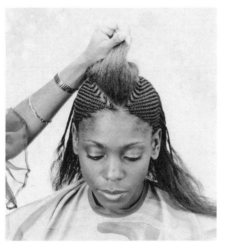

3. Braid the ends of the cornrows together then pin them flat to the head.

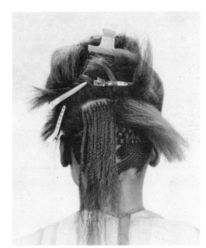

1. Section the hair from ear to ear, beneath the occipital bone.

6. Continue the "V" design throughout the top three sections.

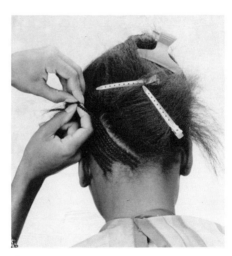

4. Cornrow the next layer down 1" longer than the natural hair.

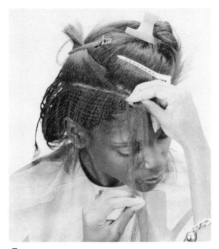

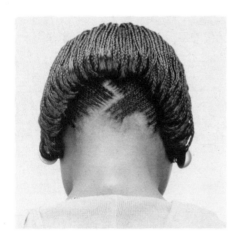

2. Cornrow the nape area upward: (if the hair is short, add a minimal amount of extension to secure the ends). To create the zig-zag part, alternate from side to side as you cornrow upward.

5. To create the wave design, make "V" partings; cornrow toward the face then angle back off the face.

7. To finish the style in a wedge back, cut the braids into an inverted "V" then bump curl the ends with a medium size curling iron.

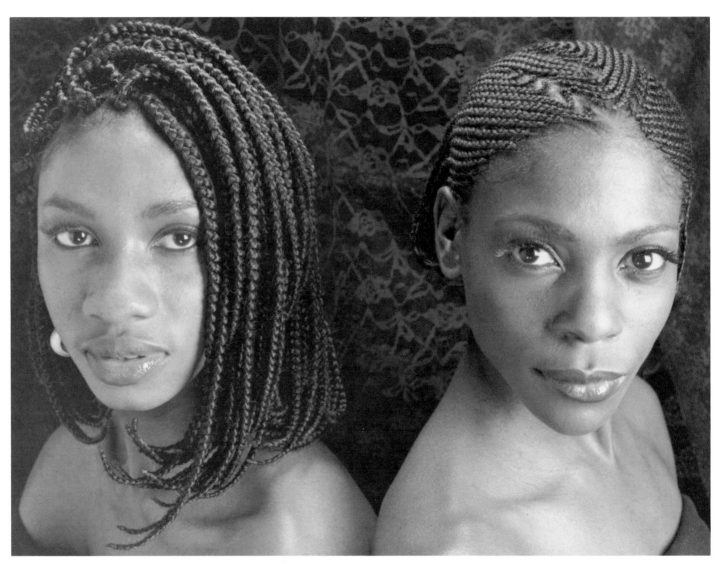

"Cultural Likeness"

"Where Style Touches Beauty"

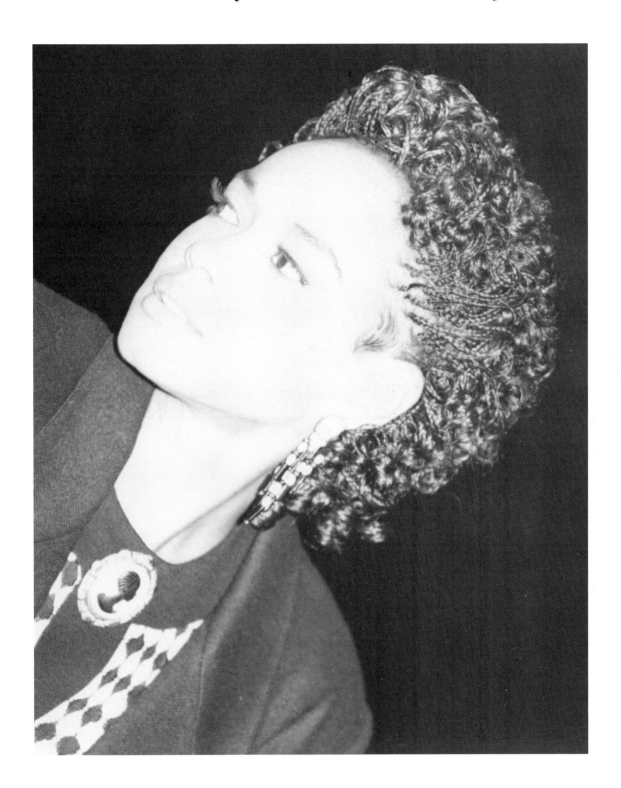

"Where Style Touches Beauty"

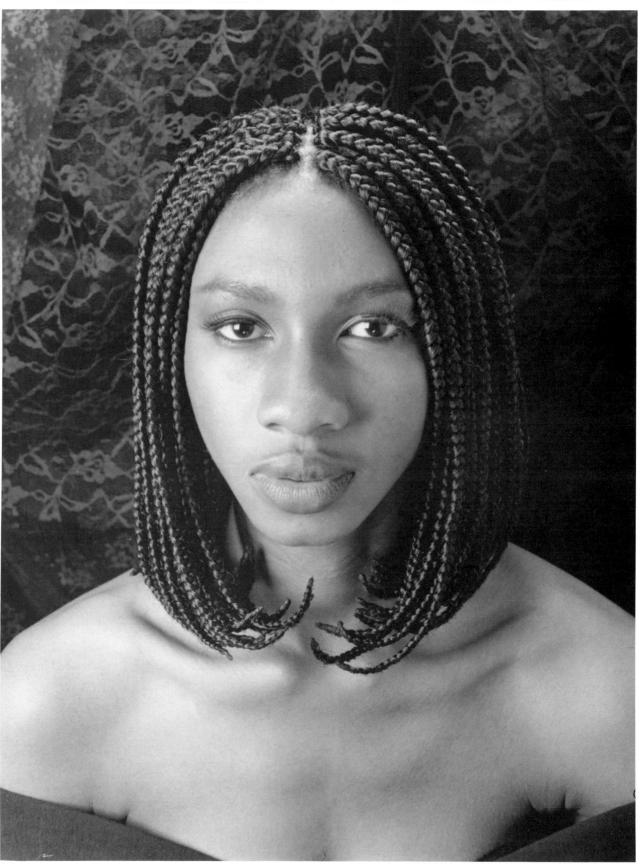

"African Bob Braids"

Tight stitch individual braids are a popular style in Western Africa. Because of its durability this style is perfect for women on the go with a life style that requires frequent shampooing and minimal after care. Our model, whose hair was thinning from chemical over processing can enjoy this style for up to 3 months in order to allow her hair to rest and rejuvenate.

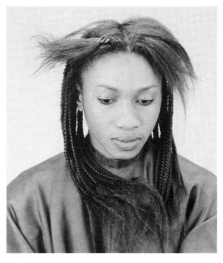

1. Begin at the back hairline. Part a 1" round section and add a thick amount of synthetic hair extension.

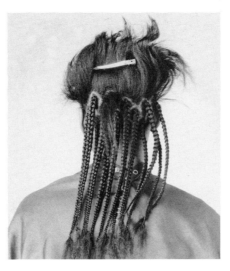

3. Braid the ends so that they taper down very narrow.

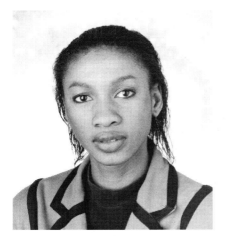

Before

Preparation: Six packs of synthetic fiber, comb, scissors, clips and butane lighter.

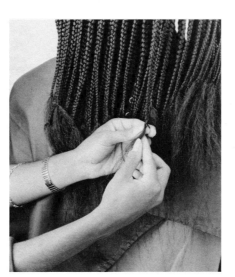

2. Make a center part. Continue braiding from the back up to the front part.

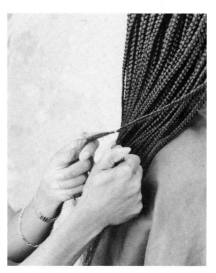

4. With a butane lighter gently burn the end of each braid to seal it closed.

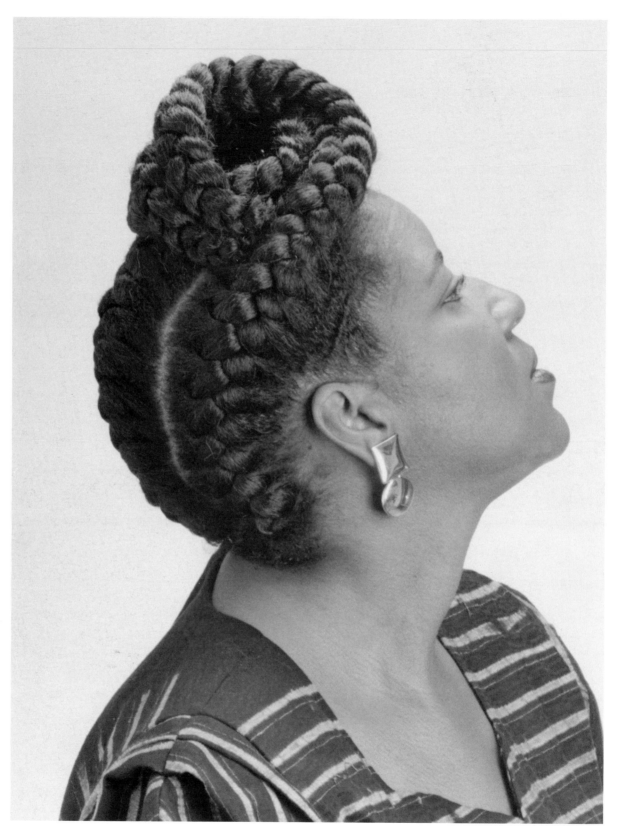

" Upper Volta"
Thick rows of African braids end in a soft, explosive sculpture..

116

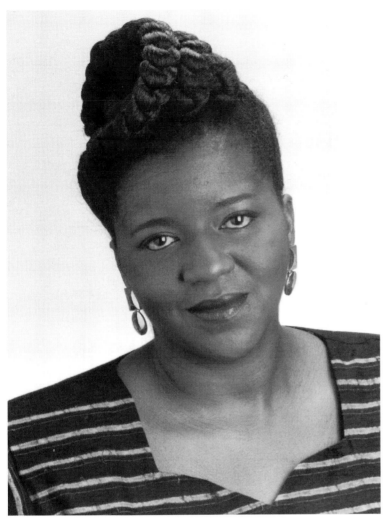

How - to:

1. Section the hair into three vertical parts.

2. Using the under hand method cornrow a thick amount of synthetic extension into each section. To seal the ends burn gently .

3. Style the braids off the forehead and pin in place with hair pins.

4. This style takes one hour to do and will last up to two weeks.

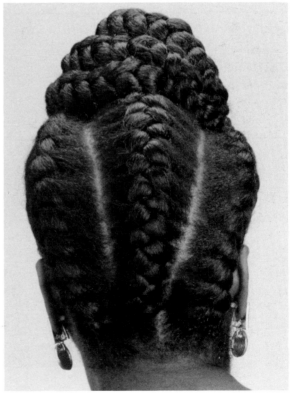

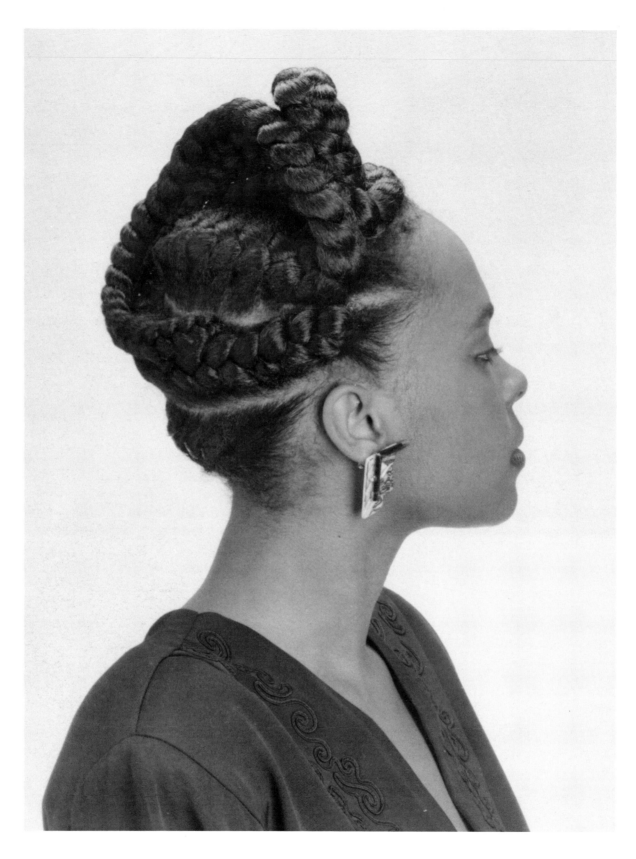

" Feathered Hat "

118

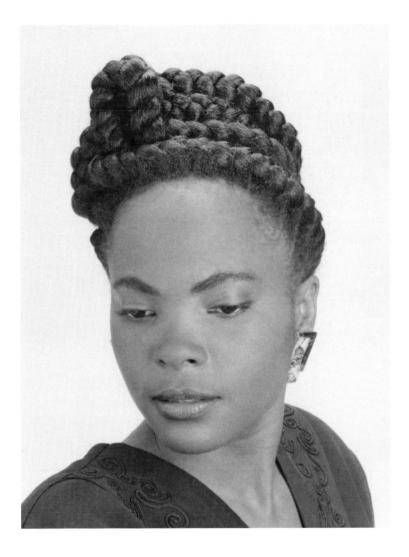

How-to:

1. Section the hair into the desired style.

2. Add a full package of hair extension to the natural hair that is pre-divided into 3 sections. Use a pack of extension per braid.

3. Incorporate the extension into the natural hair, using the under-hand braid method.

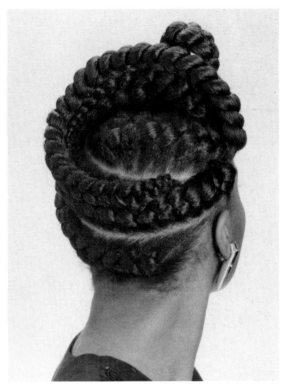

119

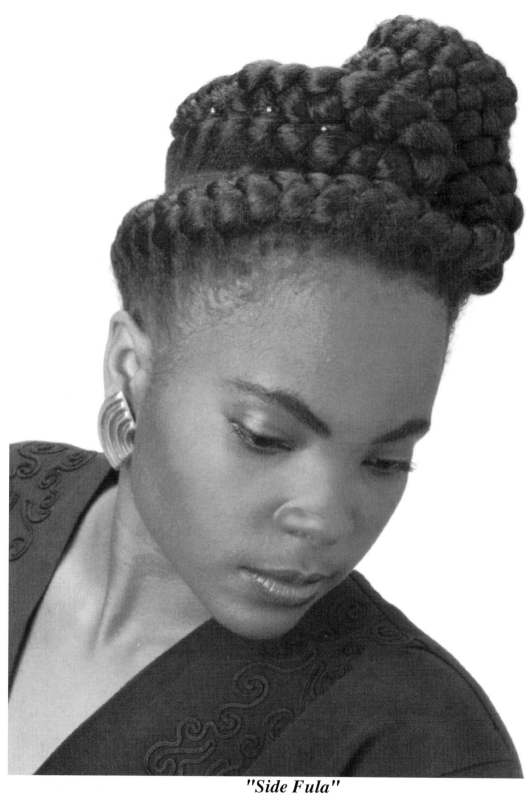

"Side Fula"

120

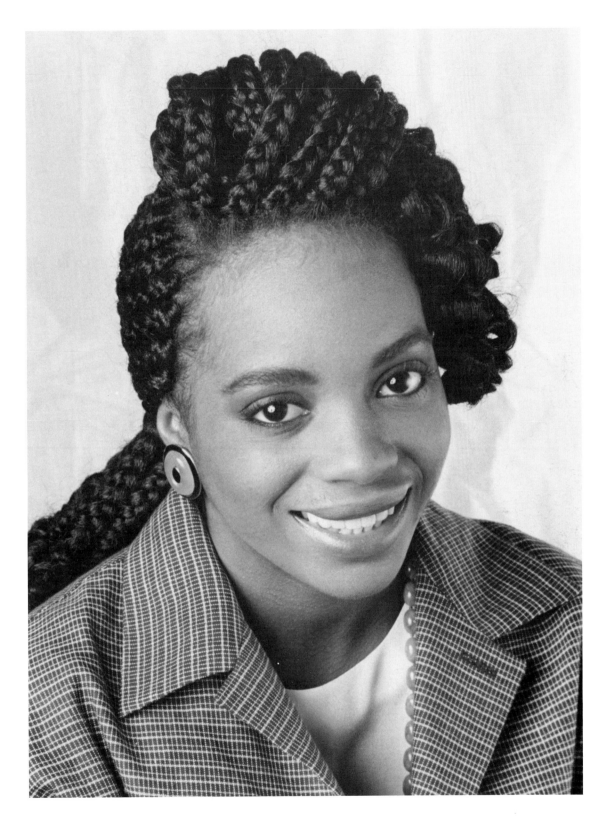

Thick braids with an African curl.

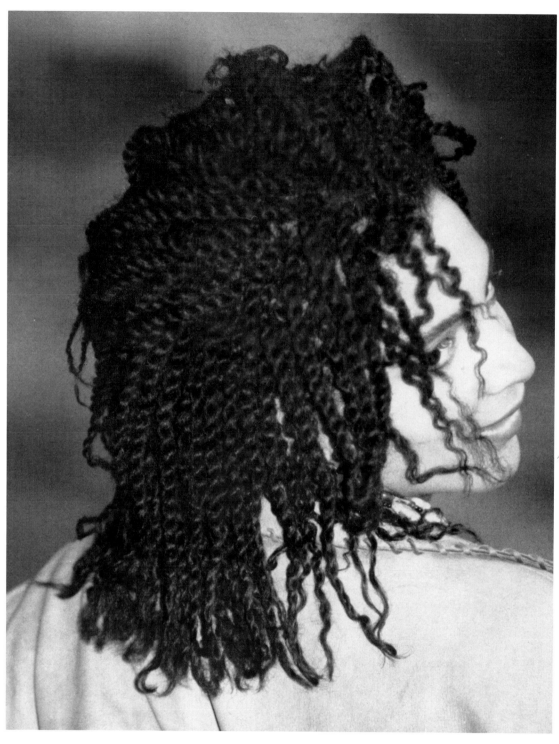

Two-strand twist are simple enough to do on yourself. Blow-dry the natural hair; then using small sections of hair, divide into two pieces. Twist the hair loosely in a criss-cross motion. The kink in the natural hair is what holds the ends together. This style can take two hours and will last at least two weeks.

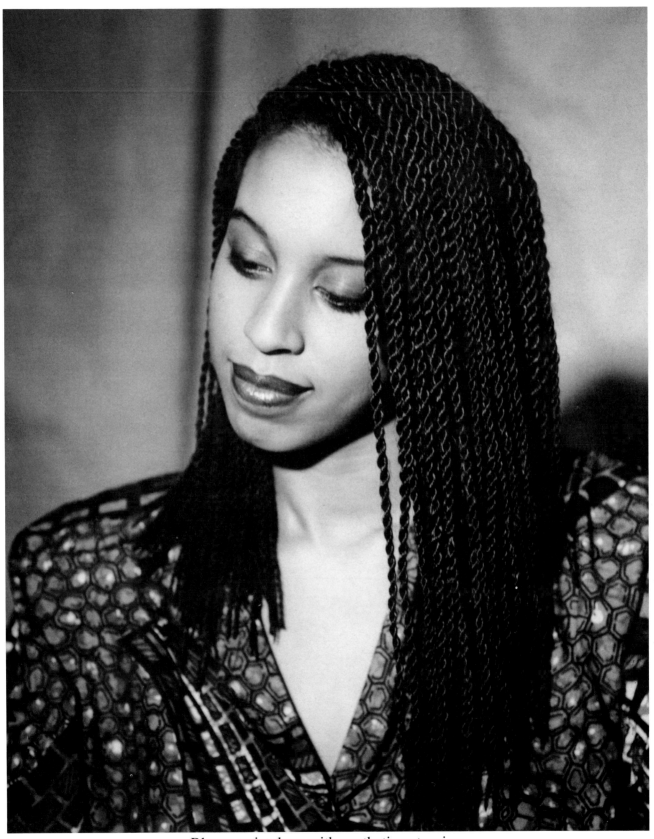

Rhasta twist done with synthetic extension.

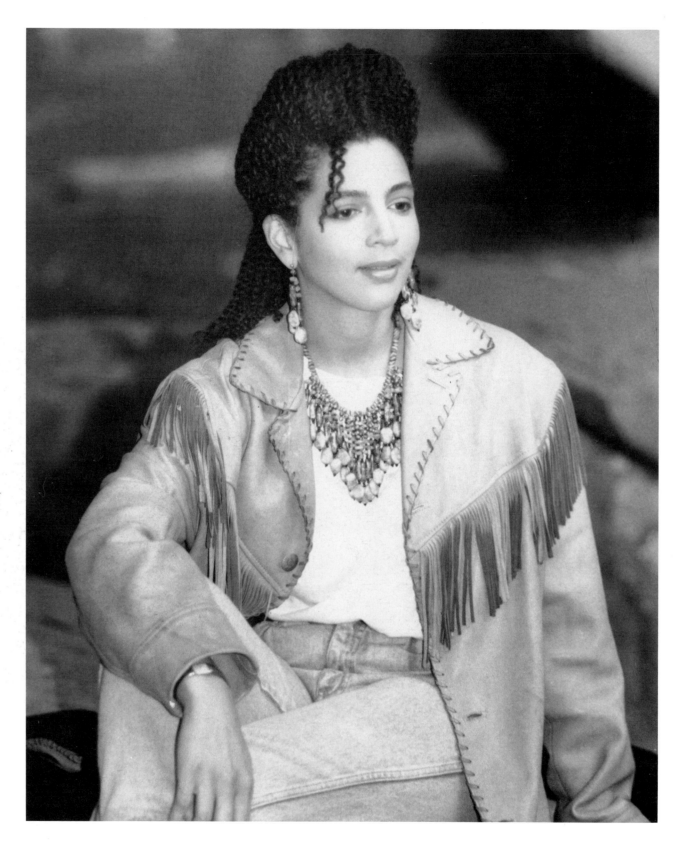

"Carefree Twist"

Two-strand twist can be worn loose or constructed into a sculpted beehive front with a hanging back.

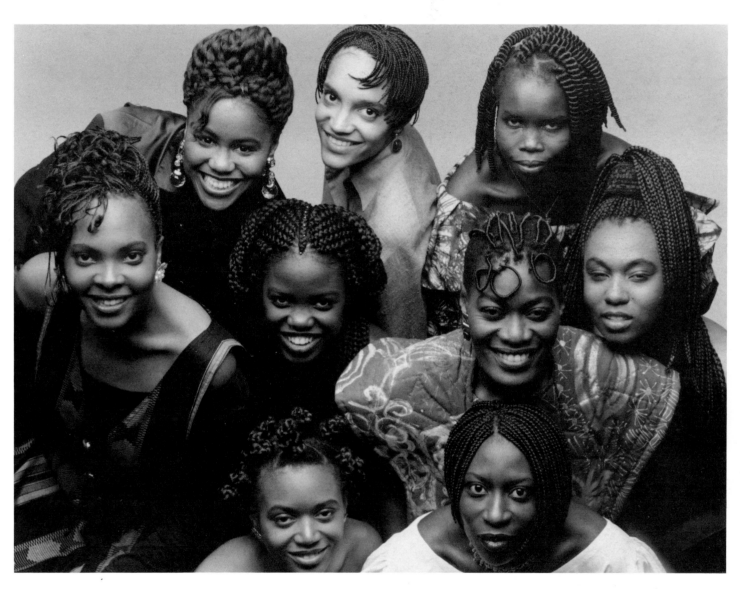

"Garden of Beauty..."

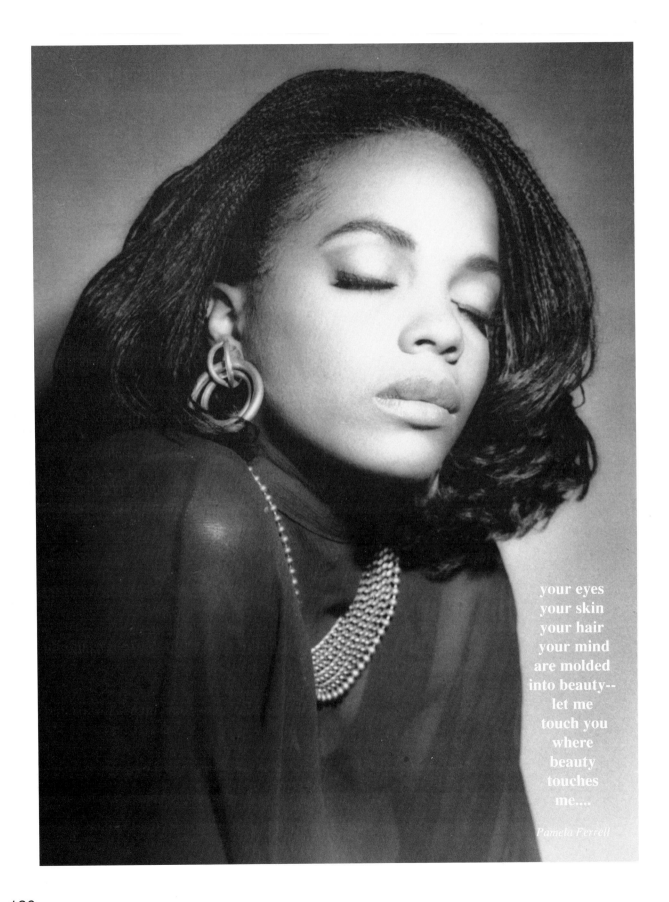

your eyes
your skin
your hair
your mind
are molded
into beauty--
let me
touch you
where
beauty
touches
me....

Pamela Ferrell

126

Special Thanks... to my beautiful clients and models.

Althea Laing
Anika Clark
Betty Entzminger
Bridget Walker
Carol Chang
Elizabeth Johnson
Erika Riggs *(pg xiv) Photo courtesy of Cosan Arts Institue*
Fatou Sambe
Gladys Thompson
Gayle George
Gail Rubin. *(page48) Photo courtesy B.L. Ochman PR, N.Y. , Hair by Pam Ferrell*
Jacqueline Onefeather Houston
Jalila Karima Mabry
Joy Mountain
Juan Laster
Judy Latta
Julia Perkins
Khady Fall
Kim Chisley
Kim Johnson
Kimberly Barnes
Leacadia Powell
Linda Lundsford
Linda Taylor
Lisa Dionne Gaskins
Lisa Harvey
Marjorline Adam *(page 61)Photo courtesy: Pivot Point's Designing Hair Additions Coursebook   Hair by Pam Ferrell*
Nancy Charles Helen
Naysha Clark
Nikki Bellamy
Njideka N. Olatunde
Pamela Dumuje
Phillip Gilliam
Sharmon Thornton
Sharon Johnson
Tanya Hill
Toinette Thompson
Toni Scott
Tracie Simmons
Triphena Johnson. *(pg 51) Photo courtesy Pivot Point, Designing Hair Additions Coursebook Hair by Ferrell*
Vanessa Washington *(page 46,47) photo courtesy B.L. Ochman PR NY,*

Hair by Pam Ferrell pg 46, 47
Mrs Viola Gibson
Wanda Frink

Photographers
Andre Richardson, Washington D.C.(Pages--cover, xi, xii, 22, 23(#1-3), 24-35, 39, 42, 44, 45, 70, 72, 74, 75, 82-112, 114-120, 125) (Cosan Arts Institute)

Irena Lukasiewicz, Chicago, Ill. (Pages--10, 49, 51, 54-63, 65-69, 73, 76-81, 113, 122-124, 126)

Diane Rubinger , N.Y, N.Y. (Pages 46-48, 121)
Al Scott, Washington D.C. (Pages. 15,17, 21, 23)
Edgar Thompson, Wash., D.C.(Pages-10, 50,52,53,64)
Kevin Tripp, Greenville, N.C. (Pages--7, 8)

Fashion Accessories and Services
African Eye Fashions, Wash. D.C (pg. 62, 63)
Sun Gallery Goldsmiths   Wash., D.C. (pg.44)
Model Agency/ Designer's Goldfinger Wash., D.C.
Make-Up/ Eric Spearman Wash., D.C.
    Sharon Richmond
    Pamela Ferrell

Assistant Hair braiders
Fatou Sambe
Tonya Raymond
Khady Fall

If I have forgotten anyone, please forgive the error.

Computer graphics, layout & design
Pamela Ferrell

Digital Imaging by Andre Richardson

For Further Reading:

Airola, Dr. Paavo; *Stop Hair Loss* Health Publishers; Phoenix, Arizona 1965-1984

Bundles Perry,A'Lelia ; Madam C. J. Walker Entrepreneur Chelsea House Publications 1991

Balch, James F.,M.D. Balch, Phyllis A. C.N.C.; *Prescription for Healing* Avery Publishing Group; Garden City Park, N.Y. 1990

Boone, Sylvia Ardyn; *Radiance from the Waters Ideals of Feminine Beauty in Mende Art*
Yale University Press 1986

Huet, Michel; *The Dance, Art and Ritual of Africa* Pantheon Publisher

Morrow, Willie; *400 Years Without a Comb* Willie Morrow; Morrows Marketing, Publishing, Research Development Corp.; San Diego, CA

Marshall Cavendish Books Unlimited (publisher) *Peoples of Africa* 58 Old Compton St., London W1V 5PA 1978

Powitt, A.H. *Hair Structure and Chemistry Simplified* Milady Publishing Corporation, N.Y. 1972 1977 1987

Sertima, Ivan Van; *Black Women in Antiquity* Transaction Publishers, New Brunswick, USA 1984

Winter, Ruth; *A Consumer's Dictionary of Cosmetic Ingredients* ; Crown Publishers, Inc. New York 1984

INDEX

Other Cornrows & Co. Products

1. ***Gallery Of Artstyles*** Full color braid style book; features over 50 braid, twist, cornrow and African curl styles. **($17.95)** *

2. ***"Thunderhead" Hair care video*** A 22-minute how-to video that demonstrates the proper shampoo, comb out, blow dry and how to cornrow the natural hair. Great for parents, teenagers and anyone that wants to know how to care for natural hair. **($32.95)** *

3. ***Care Instruction Booklet for Braid Styles***. A 12-page booklet with photos and text that shows how to shampoo and care for braided hair styles. **($2.50)** *

4. ***Cornrows & Co. Natural hair care products.*** Rosemary and Coconut shampoo, herbal conditioner and our special blend natural hair oil.

   Shampoo 8 oz. $3.99
   Conditioner 8oz. $5.99
   Hair oil 4oz. $4.99 / 8oz. $10

* All prices include domestic shipping within the Continental U.S., (Alaska, Hawaii and other countries include $5.00 for postage) Rate of exchange in U.S. Dollars

---

Wholesale prices are available to distributors, bookstores, libraries and retailers.

To order these items, send a check or money order to: *Cornrows & Co*
5401 14th St. N.W.
Washington, D.C. 20011

Call **1 800-543-3448** to place credit card orders.

Join our mailing list for future publications and seminars in your area. Make a photo copy and mail to:
Cornrows & Co **5401 14th St, N.W. Washington D.C. 20011**

Name_____

Address_____Apt#_____

City_____State_____Zip Code_____

__Mailing list only   How did you hear about this publication? ___bookstore ___magazine ___other_____

Method of payment   ___Check   ___Money order $_____(Do not send cash)
Indicate the quantity of each item:
#1_____   #2_____   #3_____   #4_____   other products_____